WOMEN IN
SHAPE

WOMEN IN
SHAPE

Published *by Boatswain Press Ltd*
Dudley House, 12 North Street
Emsworth, Hampshire PO10 7DQ
0243 377977

British Library Cataloguing in Publication Data
A catalogue record for this book is available from the British Library

ISBN 1 873432 62 3

Printed in Great Britain by Cromwell Press, Broughton Gifford, Melksham, Wiltshire

Contents

Contents – continued

STEP EXERCISES

by

Robin Gargrave

Introduction

Since its arrival in the UK, Step Training has caught the imagination of thousands of exercise enthusiasts. Many dismissed it as another 'fad' but Step Training is definitely here to stay! Why? Quite simple - it's fun and it works.

The principle of training, by stepping up and down on a raised platform, has been around for many years but manufacture of a personalised step has made possible the development of many more interesting ways of stepping up and down in the 'class' situation and in the comfort and safety of your own home.

This book aims to introduce you to Step Training – giving you the skills and knowledge to train safely and effectively and, most importantly, to have fun while you're doing it.

Before you start

Step Training, like any activity, involves an element of risk. If any of the following applies to you, you must consult your doctor before taking up this programme.

• Your doctor has said that you have a heart condition and recommends only medically supervised activity.

• You have chest pain brought on by physical activity.

• You have developed chest pain in the last month.

• You tend to lose consciousness or fall over as a result of dizziness.

• You have a bone or joint problem that could be aggravated by exercise.

• You take medication for blood pressure or a heart condition.

• You know, through your own experience or doctors advice, of any other physical reason why you should not exercise without medical supervision.

Choosing a step

There is an enormous range of steps on the market, varying in both cost and quality. You must get a step that suits your requirements but it must meet these minimum standards:–

Strong – Avoid steps that are likely to crack, split or splinter.

Stable – It must not move or slide about whilst you step. The stepping surface must be level.

Correct height – A stepping height of between four and eight inches is recommended, depending on your experience, age and level of fitness. It gets tougher as the step gets higher!

Dimension– Too small and you won't be able to perform the exercises in this book. Too large and you'll have trouble storing it.

The Y Step at 5¾" is an excellent choice. This height is enough to challenge the majority of the population and minimises the risk of injury associated with greater stepping heights. Strong and stable, it is very inexpensive at £26.00 + VAT *(at time of publication)*. It is also the only step recommended by the National Coaching Foundation.

Safety tips

In order to ensure you step safely –
• Ensure your clothing is light, comfortable and made of a material that 'breathes'.
• Wear 'trainer' type exercise shoes.
• Ensure you have enough space clear of potentially dangerous objects (furniture, toys etc). Floor should be non-slip and even.
• Never step if you have a cold, flu etc.
• If you experience pain when stepping, stop and consult your doctor immediately.
• Always drink plenty of water, before, during and after step exercise.
• Do not eat at least 2 hours before exercise.

Lifting and carrying the step

Always *'deadlift'* the step. Keep the back straight, knees in line with toes, knees over ankles, bottom a little higher than knees. Look ahead and lift, leading with the shoulders but letting the leg and bottom muscles do the work. Always lift and carry the step close to the body. To put the step down, reverse the deadlift.

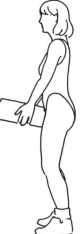

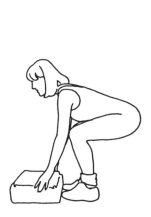

The first step

Have you noticed that the hardest thing about exercising is getting started? There are a thousand and one potential excuses and interruptions ranging from a simple 'I don't feel like it today' through 'Coronation Street looks more interesting' to the kids' arguments demanding your services as a referee! Find three hours per week (*not on consecutive days*) when you are genuinely free from distraction and be prepared to make a commitment.

Music

Step Training is more fun and more effective when done to the beat of music, but choice and speed of music is important if you are to step safely. Music speed is calculated in Beats Per Minute (*BPM*) and you can work this out by tapping your hand on the table to the beat of the music whilst looking at a watch or clock with second hands on it. Count the number of beats in a ten second count and multiply by 6 to give you the BPM. It is important that you exercise to music at the speeds recommended in this book. Specialist tapes for 'aerobics' and Step Training have the BPM of the tracks printed on the cover. It is important to choose music you like and enjoy.

Good posture position

It is important to stand and exercise with good posture. Before starting any exercises, ensure you are in the good posture position. Stand with feet shoulder width apart and slightly turned out. Pull the tummy in and tuck the bottom under slightly. Keep the shoulders relaxed and down with the knees slightly bent or 'soft'. The following body parts should now form a vertical line.

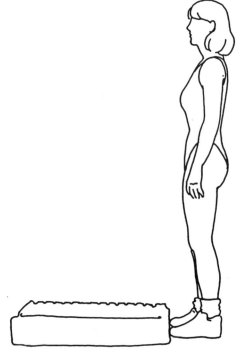

Earlobe - Shoulder - Hip - Knee - Ankle

WARM UP EXERCISES

Before starting a Step Training session always warm up for at least 10 minutes. A short period of mental and physical preparation will help you feel comfortable and lower the risk of accident or injury. The first part of the warm up is designed to warm your muscles, loosen your joints and gradually increase your heart rate. Don't do too much too soon – if you find yourself getting excessively breathless slow down and take it a bit easier. As you get fitter you will be able to warm up more vigorously.

Music

Music should be fun with a distinctive, continuous beat (124/130 BPM).

1. March on the Spot

Easy marching bringing knees up, working the arms back and forth, using just a little more effort than if walking.
Place the foot deliberately but without
crashing down. Increase effort by
taking knees a bit higher and working
arms a little more. Gradually increase
the intensity. Perform for about 1½
minutes to the beat of the music.

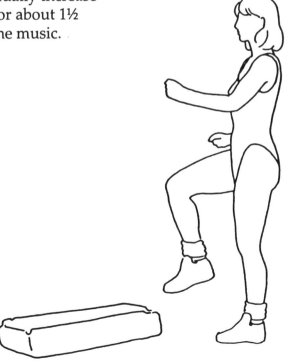

2. Plie & Arm Swings

Stand with good posture and widen the stance pointing the toes out more. Squat up and down by bending and straightening legs - not too deep. Make sure knees go out in the same direction as the feet are pointing and stay 'soft' when legs are straightened. Repeat 16 times then add arm swings in and out. Make sure you don't 'swing out' above head height. Repeat 24 times.

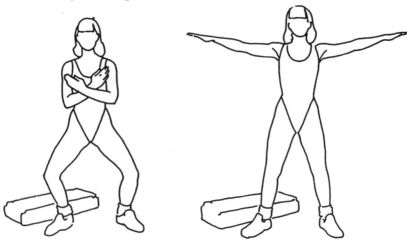

3. Side Swing Step & Neck Mobility

Take the feet wide apart and step side to side transferring your weight from one foot to the other bending the knees in the middle of the movement. Add an arm swing by taking the arms across the body in the direction of travel. Mobilise the neck by looking to the side as you travel one way and to the other as you swing back. Repeat 32 times keeping the movement flowing and gentle.

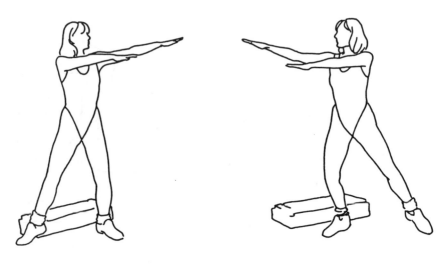

4. Side Bends

Stand with good posture and put your hands on your waist. Gently bend the upper body to the left, return to centre then bend to the right. Keep tummy pulled in and bottom under so that you don't lean forwards or back. Repeat 8 times alternating sides, ensuring the movement is controlled and comfortable.

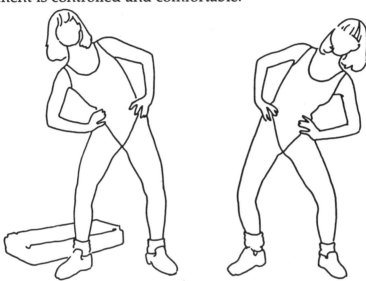

5. March & Row

March as before but with a little more vigour. Keep the arms and elbows up at shoulder height and draw them as far back as is comfortable in a 'rowing action' before pushing them out in front of you. Repeat 16 times.

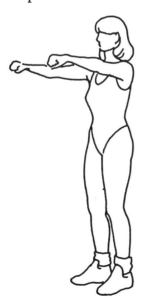
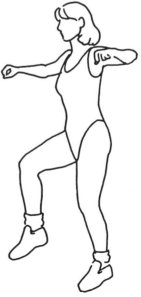

6. Trunk Twists

Stand with good posture and place the hands comfortably behind the head. 'Fix' the lower body with hips and knees facing forward. Ignore the music and slowly twist the body to one side as far as is comfortable. Return to centre. Repeat to the other side. Perform eight on each side.

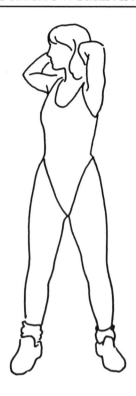

7. Knee Raise & Pull Down

Stand comfortably and lift one knee by flexing at the hip. The supporting leg should be bent slightly at the knee. Repeat on the other leg. When you feel comfortable alternating the legs, put your arms in the air and gently pull down as the knee comes up. Return the arms above the head as the knee comes down.
Repeat 24 times to the beat of the music.

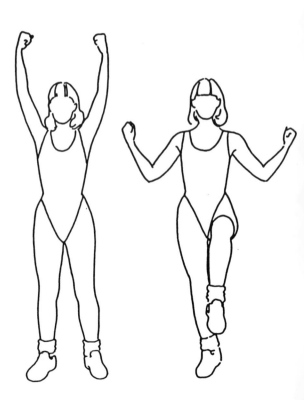

8. Hip Circles

Stand with good posture and place the hands on your hips. Keep the knees bent and the shoulders still as you describe a circle with your hips. Keep the movement flowing. Perform 8 in one direction - 8 in the other.

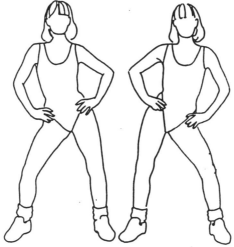

9. March & Arm Circles

March quite vigorously on the spot until you feel thoroughly warm, but (hopefully!) not puffed out. Add arm circles to really loosen the shoulders. Repeat 16 times.

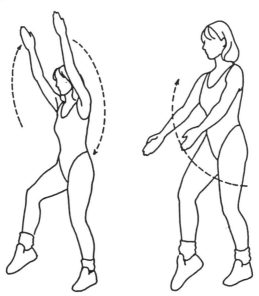

*To finish, relax the muscles and give your whole body a good shake out –
wrists, elbows, shoulders, hips, knees and ankles*

WARM UP STRETCHES

Turn the music down and don't attempt to work to the beat. These stretches will loosen the muscles and allow you to work more comfortably and efficiently and help lessen the likelihood of injury.

Technique Tips
In order to stretch safely and effectively, follow these simple guidelines:–
• Move slowly into the stretch position. When you feel the stretch hold for 9-12 seconds.
• Modify the positions so that you feel comfortable. Experience the stretch in the target area.
• Experience the stretch as a mild tension. Never stretch to the point of pain.
• Breathe regularly and rhythmically throughout.

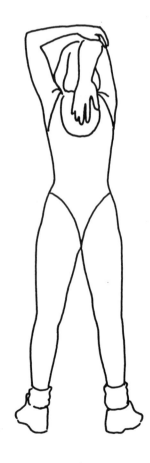

1. Back of the Arm
            (Triceps)
Stand comfortably with good posture. Drop one arm down the back behind your head and relax that arm. Apply gentle pressure downwards and across with the opposite hand until you experience the stretch, then hold.

2. Chest Stretch

(Pectorals)
Stand comfortably with good posture. Link your fingers in front of your body then slowly lift the arms above the head until you experience the stretch, then hold.

3. Front of Shoulder & Upper Chest

(Anterior Deltoid & Pectoralis Minor)
Stand with good posture. Link the fingers behind the body, then slowly lift the arms and squeeze the shoulder blades together until you experience the stretch, then hold.

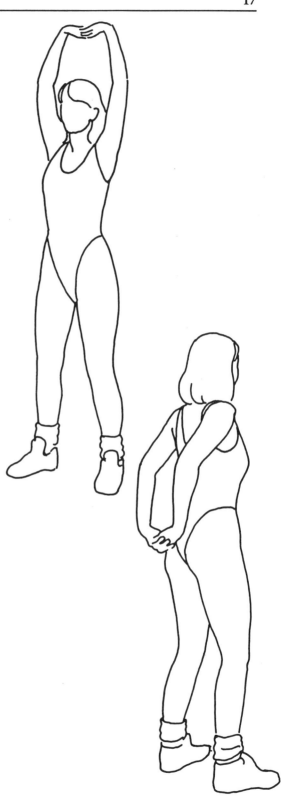

4. Side Stretch

(Obliques, Pectorals,
Latissimus Dorsi)
Stand with the feet com-
fortably wider than your
normal stance. Place one
hand on the thigh for support and raise the other one
in the air. Slowly flex to
one side, keeping the hips
central and avoiding any
forward or backward 'twist'
until you experience the
stretch, then hold. Return
to the start position under
control and repeat on the
other side.

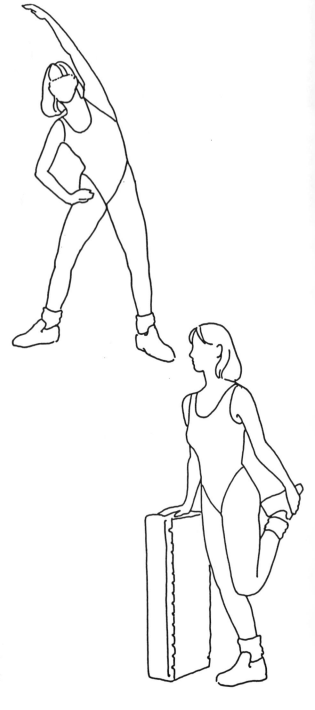

5. Front of Thigh

(Quadricep)
Using your step on its end
to assist with balance, bend
at the knee. Take hold of
your instep and pull the heel
gently towards your bot-
tom and push the hip
forward until you experi-
ence the stretch, then hold.
Maintain an upright pos-
ture with the hips facing
forward and the legs parallel. Slightly bend the
supporting knee. Repeat
on the opposite leg.

6. Calf Stretch

(Soleus & Gastrocnemius)
Place one foot wholly on the centre of the step with the knee above the ankle *(toes & hips facing forward).* The foot of the straight rear leg also points forward. The foot should only be far enough back to get the heel down on the floor comfortably.   Slowly take the weight forward and slightly flex the leading knee.   At the same time, press the rear heel into the floor until you experience the stretch, then hold. Repeat with the other leg leading.

7. Lower Calf Stretch

(Soleus)
Keep the same position but bring the rear leg closer to the step and bend the knee. Gently let your weight come down to help bend the rear knee further until you experience the stretch.   Then hold. Repeat with the other leg leading.

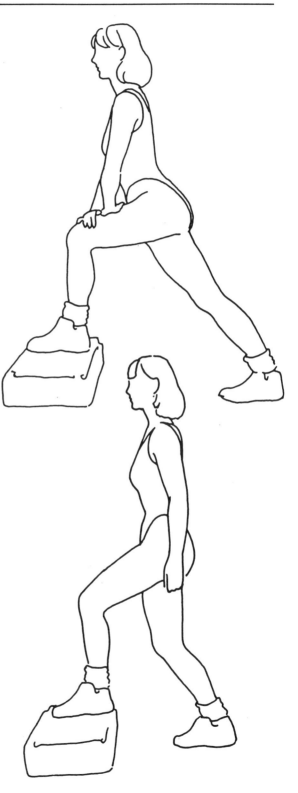

8. Front of Hip Stretch
(Iliacus & Psoas Major)
Keep the same position. Lift the heel of the rear leg. This will allow you to tuck your pelvis right under. Push the hip of the rear leg gently forward until you experience the stretch, then hold. Repeat with the other leg leading.

9. Back of Thigh Stretch
(Hamstrings)
Keep the same position but straighten the leading leg. Using your arms on the thigh of the rear leg to support your weight, slowly lean forward at the hips, looking ahead to keep the back straight with tummy in until you experience the stretch, then hold. Repeat with the other leg leading.

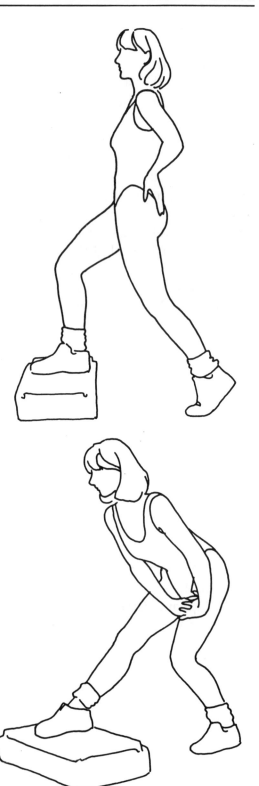

10. Groin Stretch *(Adductors)*

Stand to one side of your step. Place your whole foot on the step. The toes should point to the diagonally opposite corner of the step. Keeping the weight over the other leg *(support with the arms if necessary)* gradually ease the foot on the step to the side and away from the body until you experience the stretch, then hold. Repeat with the other leg leading.

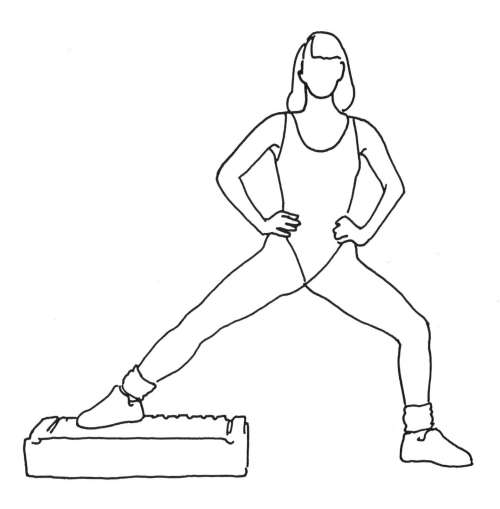

Second warm up

The warm up stretches will have cooled you down a little, so spend at least two minutes getting warm again. Bring the warm up music volume back up and spend 2 minutes getting familiar with your step. March on the top of it, walk round it and tap the top of it with alternate heels and toes. Gradually increase the vigour and range of your exercises over the two minutes until you feel thoroughly warm and confident about being on the step.

AEROBIC STEP TRAINING

Step Training is excellent for improving the efficiency of your heart, lungs and circulatory system. It should be rhythmic, moderate intensity and employ the large muscle groups in the legs. Regular aerobic training has been shown to have many health benefits including reduced risk of coronary heart disease. It can also *(in conjunction with a sensible healthy, balanced diet)*, make a significant contribution to fat loss and weight control. You should be able to step continuously and rhythmically without feeling undue fatigue. You should feel you're getting a workout but not feel too puffed to hold a conversation while stepping!

Technique Tips

It is important you step with good technique in order to maximise the safety, effectiveness and enjoyment of your workout. Follow these simple guidelines:
• Step with the whole foot on the stepping surface.
• Always step to the centre of the step.
• On the 'up' step extend your leg but don't lock the knee joint.
• On the 'down' step make sure you land close to the step on the ball of the foot, lowering your heel to the floor, keeping your knees slightly flexed.
• Keep knees aligned with feet and use smooth, controlled movements.
• Avoid movements that travel forward and down off the step.
• Don't step up or down with your back toward the step.
• Maintain good upright posture with shoulders relaxed and the tummy firm.

These tips apply to *all* the step patterns described.

The Aerobic Circuit

Perform all the exercises in the order shown – this constitutes 1 'circuit'. Master the leg work before attempting to add the arm lines – these require much greater co-ordination. Start with just 20 seconds on each exercise, rest for 10 seconds before proceeding to the next exercise. As you get fitter this will feel more comfortable and you will be able to progress to the next stage using the following guidelines. Only progress if you can manage the stage you are on comfortably.

Stage 1	*30 seconds work*	*10 seconds rest*	*Circuit x 1*
Stage 2	*30 seconds work*	*5 seconds rest*	*Circuit x 1*
Stage 3	*30 seconds work*	*No rest*	*Circuit x 1*
Stage 4	*20 seconds work*	*5 seconds rest*	*Circuit x 2*
Stage 5	*30 seconds work*	*No rest*	*Circuit x 2*
Stage 6	*40 seconds work*	*No rest*	*Circuit x 2*
Stage 7	*30 seconds work*	*5 seconds rest*	*Circuit x 3*
Stage 8	*30 seconds work*	*No rest*	*Circuit x 3*
Stage 9	*40 seconds work*	*No rest*	*Circuit x 3*
Stage 10	*50 seconds work*	*No rest*	*Circuit x 3*

If you wish to progress beyond this, 1 minute on each step pattern, 3 times round the circuit, gives you a 30 minute workout – you can consider yourself an advanced performer!

What is 'Rest'?

Don't sit down! Keep walking gently on the spot until you are ready to tackle the next step pattern. 'Rest' any time you feel like it. You should always feel comfortable. If you feel fatigue in the upper body or you lose rhythm or coordination, 'rest' by dropping out the arm lines whilst continuing with the basic step pattern.

Music

Music should be motivating, rhythmic and with a steady continuous beat (118-122 BPM). Have enough music so that you won't have to stop and change the tape or record.

Step Pattern 1   *Basic Up & Biceps Curl*

Legs
Start facing the step at the centre:
• Step up right
• Step up left and take the weight
• Step down right
• Step down left and lightly tap the toes. This will enable the left
to lead.   In this way you can alternate leading leg.

Arms
• As you step up bend at the elbows, keeping the upper arms still
and draw the forearms towards the shoulders.
• As you step down lower the forearms under control to the start
position.

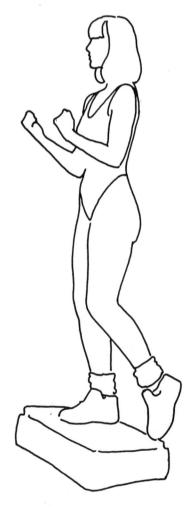

Step Pattern 2 *Basic Down & Pec Dec*

Legs

Start by standing on top of the step at the centre:

• Step back off the step with the right keeping the knee of the left over the ankle.

• Step down left and take the weight.

• Step up right and lightly tap the left toes enabling the left to lead down.

In this way you can alternate leading legs.

Arms

At the start position your upper arms are pointing directly forward at shoulder height. Bent elbows mean the lower arms are pointed towards the ceiling.

• As you step down take the upper arms out to the side of your body, maintaining a right angle at the elbow.

• As you step up return to the start position and try to squeeze your forearms together.

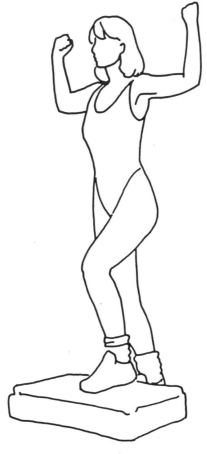

Step Pattern 3   *V Step & Rotators*

Legs

Start facing the step at the centre:

• Step up wide with the right turning the toes out slightly to point to the right top corner of the step.

• Step up wide with the left leg pointing the toes to the top left corner of the step and take the weight.

• Step down right to the centre (toes now facing forward) and take the weight.

• Step down left to the centre. Tap lightly with the left which then leads the same step to the left.

In this way you can alternate leading legs.

Arms

Shoulders are loose and low, elbows remain slightly bent throughout.

• As you step up right, push the shoulders forward and rotate the arms inward leading with the elbows.

• As you step across left, draw the shoulders back and open the arms by tucking the elbows in. Repeat to every beat of the music.

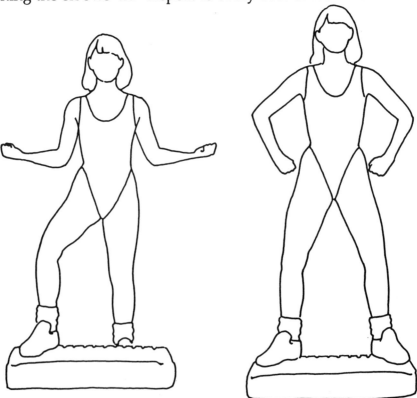

Step Pattern 4

Turn Step & Arm Sweep

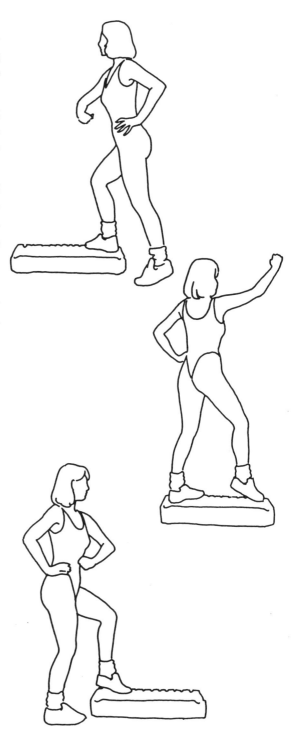

Legs

Start at the right hand corner of the step facing the diagonally opposite corner (left):

• Step on with the right with the toes facing the diagonally opposite corner (left).

• Step across with the left to the other end of the step and land with the toes facing the diagonally opposite corner (right).

• Step down with the right, tap the left which becomes the leading leg for the turn step back to the start position.

In this way you can alternate leading legs.

NB: As you turn, ensure the heel of the leading leg comes up slightly and that the hips, knees and toes are always facing the same direction and turning at the same time. Avoid any rotational force on the knee joint.

Arms

• As you step and turn, take the same arm as leading leg and sweep it in a long, controlled motion across the body and away at shoulder height.

Step Pattern 5

Alternate Step/Knee Lift & Pec Deck

Legs
Start facing the step at the centre:
• Step up right.
• Draw left knee up under control to hip height.
• Step down with the left.
• Step down with the right and take the weight. This will enable the left to lead. In this way you can alternate leading legs.

Arms
• As the knee comes up fully, draw the elbows together at chest height with the upper arms pointing to the ceiling.
• As you step down, draw the elbows back, keeping the arms at shoulder height.

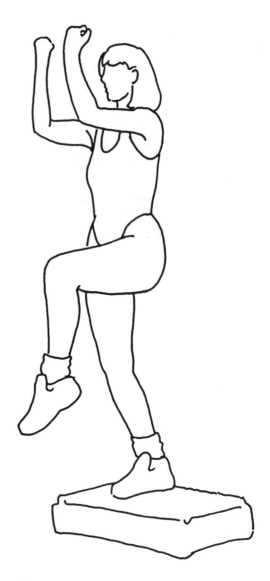

NB: Can be performed at double time, i.e. on the 'down' as well as the 'up' but ensure the movements are smooth and controlled throughout.

Step Pattern 6   *Alternate Corner Leg Curl & Lateral Raise*

Legs

Start opposite the centre of the step facing the top left corner:

• Step up right towards left hand corner. Bend the left knee drawing the heel towards the bottom. Step down left

• Step down right and turn towards top right corner. This will enable the left leg to lead.

In this way you can travel to opposite corners and alternate leading legs.

Arms

• As the leg curls, raise the arms out to the side of the body to the height of the ears.

• As you step down, return arms to the side of the body.

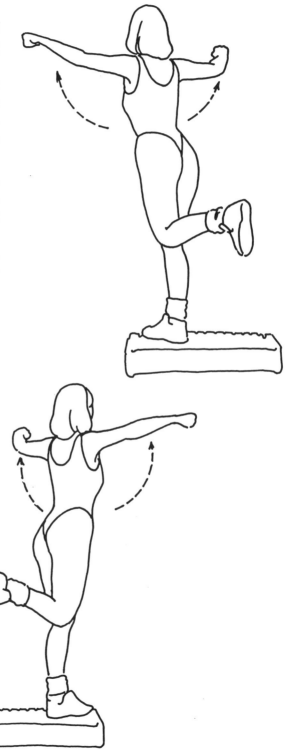

Step Pattern 7   *Lunge & Triceps Extension*

Legs
Start by standing on top of the
step at the centre:
• Step back left keeping the
weight over the right leg, knee
over ankle. Lightly tap the
toes of the left foot keeping the
heel off the floor.
• Bring the left back up and
take the weight. This enables
the right to step back and
lightly toe tap.
In this way you can alternate
leading legs.
NB: As you tap back, flex for-
ward slightly at the hips to keep
the back straight. Keep tummy
and back muscles firm to main-
tain good posture.

Arms
Start with the elbows flexed
and pushed behind you with
the shoulder blades drawn together:
• As one foot taps back extend
the elbows until the arms are
straight.
• As the foot comes back onto
the step bend the elbows fully.
• Repeat for other leg.
NB: Keep elbows behind the line
of the back throughout. The upper
arms do not move. This is a tiring
step - use with care. At the first
sign of discomfort stop and rest.

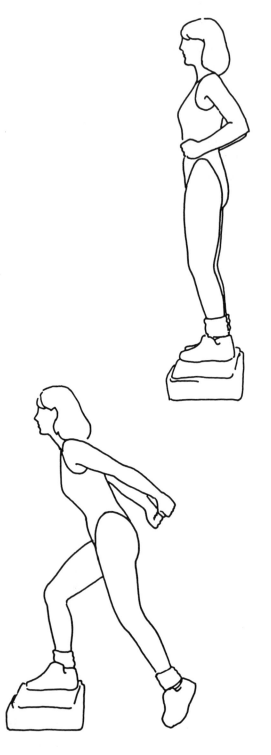

Step Pattern 8

Straddle Up & Upright Row

Legs
Start by standing astride the step length-ways with the knees slightly flexed in line with the toes which should be slightly turned out:
• Step up right, with toes facing forward
• Step up left, toes forward. Take the weight on the left.
• Step down right, toes pointing slightly out. Ankles over knees in line with toes, knees slightly bent. Take the weight on the right.
• Step down left and lightly tap the toes. This enables the left leg to lead.
In this way you can alternate leading legs.

Arms
• As you step up, pull your arms up the body, leading with the elbows. The arms stay close to the body throughout.
• As you step down, lower the arms to the start position.

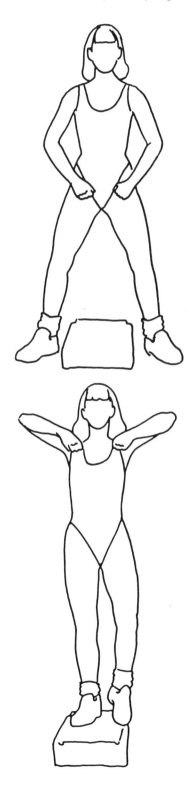

Step Pattern 9   *Over The Top & Arm Circles*

Legs

Start by standing next to the step with the step lengthways:

• Side step up right to beyond the mid-line of the step.

• Side step up left. Take the weight on the left leg.

• Side step down right away from the step leaving room for your left foot. Take the weight on your right leg.

• Side step down left and tap the toes. This enables you to side step back leading with the left.

In this way you can alternate leading legs.

Arms

• With elbows slightly bent, circle the arms across the front of the body in the direction of travel.

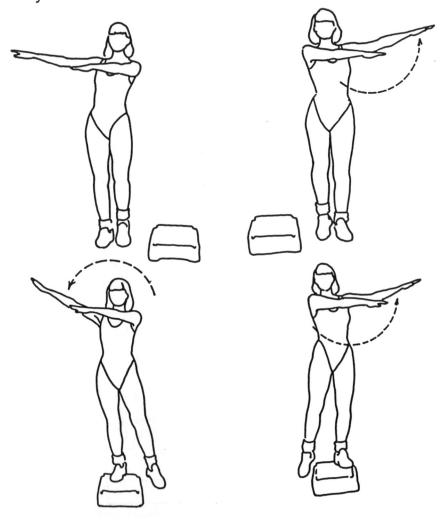

Step Pattern 10   *Straddle Down & Shoulder Press*

Legs

Start by standing on top of the step with the step lengthways:

• Step down left, turning toes out slightly, keeping ankle over knee which should be in line with toes. Step down with the knee slightly bent. Take the weight.

• Step down right with knee and ankle in the same alignment. You should now be 'astride' the step. Take the weight on the right leg.

• Step up left. Toes, knees and hips now face forward.

• Step up right to lightly tap the toes. This enables you to step down leading with the right.

In this way you can alternate leading legs.

Arms

Start with the elbows bent. Fingers touching shoulders:

• As you step down, push both arms into the air above the head.

• As you step up, lower the arms under control to the start position.

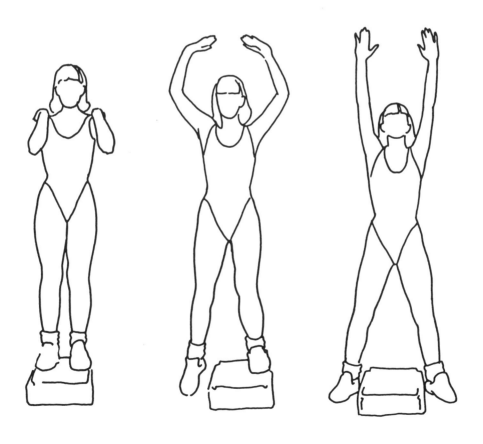

COOLDOWN

Never suddenly stop vigorous exercise. Always spend 4-5 minutes gradually lowering the intensity of the exercise. This will aid recovery, gradually returning your heart and breathing rate to near normal levels.

All the exercises have been described earlier in this book. Perform in the recommended order.

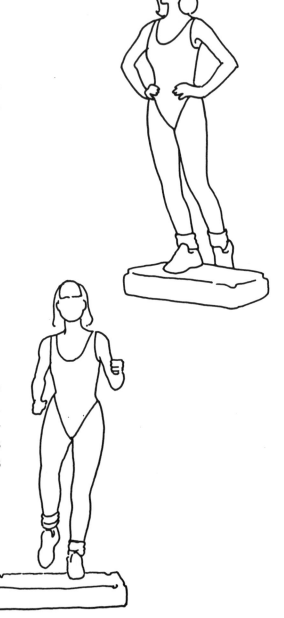

1. Basic Up
(1 minute 30 seconds)
As for Step Pattern 1 but don't use the arms. Rest the hands on hips. Breathe and relax.

2. Vigorous March
(30 seconds)
As for Warm up Exercise 1 performed on top of the step but start vigorously and gradually make it less vigorous by lowering the arms and not lifting the knees as high.

3. Side Swing Step
(30 seconds)
As for Warm up Exercise 3 but leave out neck mobility. Gradually decrease the distance between the feet and lower the arm swings.

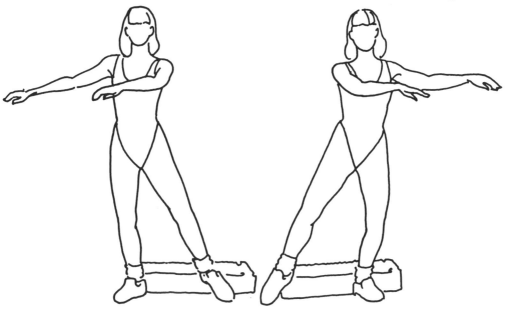

4. Plie & Arm Swings
(30 seconds)
As for Warm up Exercise 2 but don't bend the knees as much. Relax the shoulders on the arm swings and gradually lower the height of the arms.

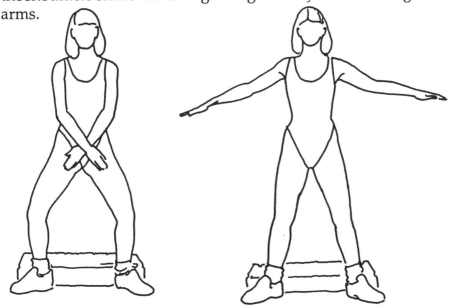

5. Walk on the Spot

Walk on the spot, gently shaking your arms and occasionally kicking out your legs until you feel fully recovered. Finish with some gentle side bends (Warm up Exercise 4) and Hip circles (Warm up Exercise 8). Now shake out and get ready for some muscle fitness work.

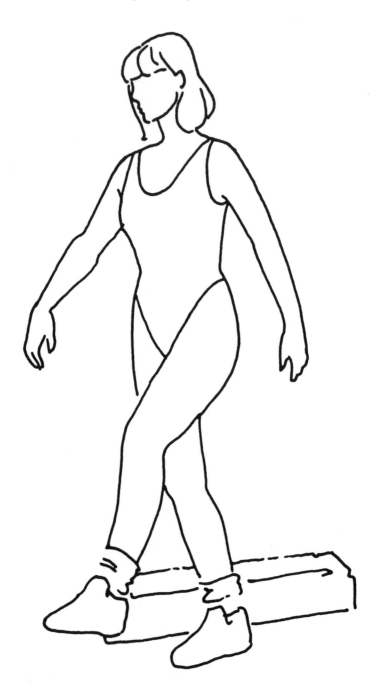

MUSCULAR STRENGTH & ENDURANCE
STEP TRAINING

These exercises will help improve your 'muscle fitness' and contribute to toning your body, improving your posture and making daily tasks seem easier.

Technique Tips

It is import you perform these exercises with good technique in order to maximise the safety, effectiveness and enjoyment of your workout. Follow these simple guidelines:
- Ensure exercise position is comfortable.   Place a mat or carpet under any body part in contact with the step or floor.
- Perform exercises through the fullest possible range of movement.
- Perform slowly and under control
- Feel fatigue in the target muscles. Never exercise to the point of pain.
- Breathe regularly and rhythmically throughout.
- Rest between sets of exercises until muscles feel fully recovered.

The MSE Circuit

Perform **all** the exercises in the order shown. One single complete exercise is called a *'repetition'*. A group of repetitions is known as a *'set'*. Only perform enough repetitions to feel the onset of fatigue in the target muscles. As you get fitter you will be able to perform more repetitions and sets of exercises and be able to progress through the stages recommended below. Only progress when you can manage all the recommended repetitions and sets comfortably.

	Position	*Reps*	*Sets*
Stage 1	A	5-10	1
Stage 2	A	10-15	1
Stage 3	A	15-20	1
Stage 4	A	20-25	1
Stage 5	A	15-20	2
Stage 6	A	20-25	2
Stage 7	B	10-15	2
Stage 8	B	15-20	2
Stage 9	B	15-20	3
Stage 10	B	20-25	3

Music
Music should have a strong, prominent beat (118-120 BPM).

MSE Exercise 1

Press-up   *(Chest & Arms - Pectorals, Triceps)*
• Hands 1½ x shoulder width apart on the step, fingers facing forward.
• Shoulders over hands
• Bend at elbows and lower nose between hands keeping elbows out to the side and back straight.
• Push up to straighten the arms without locking the elbow joint.

Position A

Knees under Hips

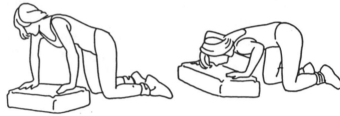

Position B

Keep the back straight
with knees bent throughout

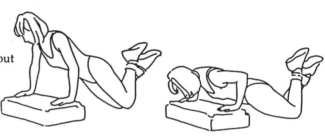

MSE Exercise 2

Curl-ups   *(Tummy - Rectus Abdominus, Internal/External Obliques)*
• Place feet comfortably on the step and lie on your back with knees and hips bent.
• Place one hand on the thigh and support the head with the other hand. Pull the tummy in.
• Without twisting, curl the spine off the floor to reach the hand on the thigh towards the knee.
• Lower under control to the start position.

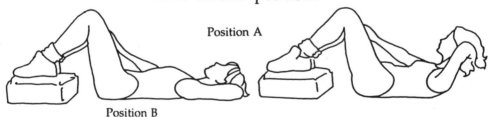

Position A

Position B

Both hands support the head. Never 'pull' on the head

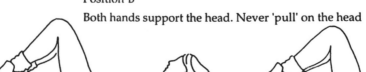

MSE Exercise 3
Back Extension   *(Back - Erector Spinae)*
• Lie comfortably face down on the step with trunk and hips supported.
• Keep looking down and slowly lift the chest from the step - keep toes on the floor at all times.
• Lower under control to the start position.

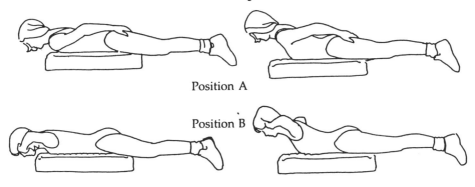

Position A

Position B

MSE Exercise 4
Hip Extension   *(Gluteals)*
• Lie comfortably face down on the step with your head and hips supported.
• Keeping hips in contact with step, lift one leg in the air as far as is comfortable.
• Lower under control to the start position. Repeat on the opposite leg.

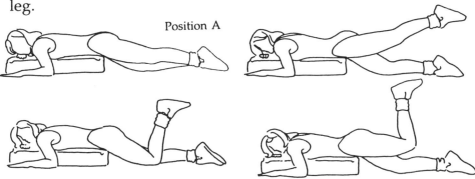

Position A

Position B Keep knee of the lifted leg bent throughout the exercise

After your MSE Circuit, stand up carefully and give your body a gentle shake out. Walk around for a minute or two until you feel loose and ready to stretch.

COOLDOWN STRETCHES

Always end your step workout with these stretching exercises to help relax the muscles you have been working and return them to their normal length. They also reduce the likelihood of immediate post exercise stiffness and may contribute to improved flexibility. This will allow you to move your limbs freely through a greater range of movement and help improve posture. Stretching aids more skilful movement and generally reduces the risk of injury.

Technique Tips

In order to stretch safely and effectively follow these simple guidelines.

• Move slowly into the stretch position. When you feel the stretch, hold for 15-25 seconds.

• Modify the positions so that you feel comfortable. Place a mat or carpet under any body part in contact with the floor or the step.

• Experience the stretch in the target area.

• Experience the stretch as a mild tension. Never stretch to the point of pain.

• Breathe regularly and rhythmically.

Music

Music should be relaxing – no dominant beat.

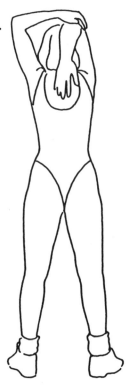

1. Back of the Arm *(Triceps)*

Stand with good posture. Drop one arm down the back behind your head and relax that arm. Apply gentle pressure downwards and across with the opposite hand until you experience the stretch. Repeat on the opposite arm.

2. Chest *(Pectorals)*
Stand comfortably with good posture. Link the fingers in front of your body then slowly lift the arms above the head until you experience the stretch, then hold.

3. Calf Stretch *(Soleus &*
Gastrocnemius)
Stand away from the step. Take one leg forward and place the toes on the edge of the step with the heel on the floor. Straighten the leading leg while bending the rear leg, keeping the body upright. When comfortable and stable with toes pointing forward, gently straighten the rear leg until you experience a stretch in the calf of the leading leg then hold. Repeat on the opposite leg.

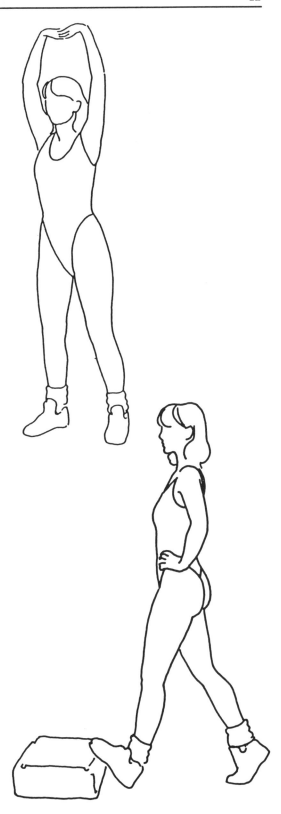

4. Lower Calf   *(Soleus)*
Same position as calf stretch but keep the knee of the leading leg bent. Straighten the knee of the rear leg until you experience the stretch in the calf of the leading leg then hold. Repeat on the opposite leg.

5. Back of Thigh Stretch
               (Hamstrings)
Lie comfortably on your back with your head and bottom supported, knees bent, feet flat on the floor. Pull one knee into the chest and gradually straighten the leg, supporting behind the calves or thigh with the hands. Keeping the leg straight, gently move the leg closer to the body until you experience the stretch, then hold. Repeat on the opposite leg.

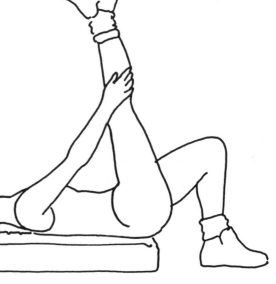

6. Inner Thigh
(Adductors)

Sit on the step and bring the soles of your feet together. Hold the ankles and gently push the knees down until you experience the stretch, then hold.

7. Front of Leg
(Quadriceps)

Lie face down on the step with your trunk and thighs supported. Head supported on one arm. Bend the knee of one leg and draw the heel towards your bottom. Hold the instep and gently pull the heel towards the bottom. At the same time push the hip into the step until you experience the stretch, then hold. Repeat on opposite leg. An easier version is achieved lying on your side.

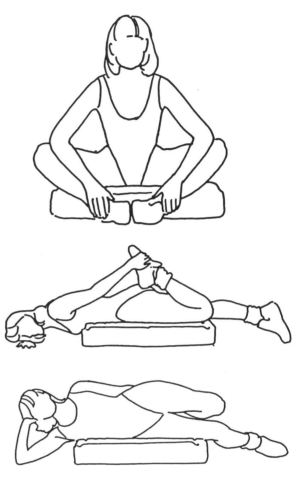

8. Front of Hip Stretch
(Illiacus & Psoas Major)

Stand up close to the step and place one foot on it. Bend the back knee, raising the heel and tuck the pelvis under pushing the hip forward until you feel a stretch at the front hip of the rear leg, then hold. Repeat with the opposite leg leading.

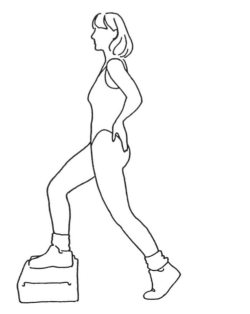

WAKE UP

Brilliant! You've completed your programme!

Put on some fun music and dance around the room for a few minutes. It will liven you up and put you in the mood to face anyone or anything. Plus the neighbours will think you're raving mad! Who cares? – you've done well. Treat yourself to a cool bath or shower and look forward to the next session.

I hope you enjoyed these exercises. If you feel you've got the basics and want to go further, why not try –

• *Step into Shape* – A Y Plan Step Exercise Video featuring Chris Smith, Jean Ann Marnoch and Paula Hamilton.

• A local Step Class – but do make sure your teacher is qualified. London Central YMCA now run a training and assessment programme for Step Teachers. For further details telephone 071-580-2989.

REGAIN YOUR FIGURE AFTER CHILDBIRTH

by

Jill Gaskell

Introduction

For many women, having a baby is one of the greatest moments of their life. However, as the initial euphoria wears off, it becomes obvious that getting your body back into shape is going to require more than just a high degree of hope.

This will help you restore your figure by providing expert guidance and a series of safe and effective exercises which are easy and quick to perform. The exercises are preceded by general advice for exercise in the postnatal period, and an insight into the major physiological changes that occurred during pregnancy and how these affect your getting back into shape afterwards. For ease, the baby is referred to as 'him' throughout.

When can I start to exercise?

You can never start too soon and one or two exercises can even be commenced on day one. The sooner you start the better, as these exercises will also enhance the way you feel. Often we all have the greatest of intentions to exercise and regain our figure following pregnancy but soon find the demands of a newborn baby take over. Whilst it is important to capitalise on this desire from the word go, you should also be realistic and not overdo it. Your body needs time to adjust to caring for, and possibly feeding, a new born baby. Attempts to do too much too soon will be detrimental to your recovery and could affect your baby.

Follow the schedule suggested in the gentle postnatal programme 'one' for the first 6 weeks and remember that little – and often – is the key to sucess. Some time after this you can, and should, look to increase the amount of exercise you do – the postnatal programme 'two' will provide an effective but gradual progression. Before starting this or any other more comprehensive exercise programme however, you must check with your medical practitioner that it is all right for you to progress. The 6 week postnatal checkup is an ideal opportunity for this.

Following a caesarean section, recovery is a little slower than that of mothers who had a normal delivery. The sequence of exercises outlined in the postnatal programmes are suitable for both but, if you had a caesarean section or a particulary difficult birth, you should take an even more gentle approach.

When is it safe for me to go swimming?

Swimming is an excellent form of exercise for you as it does not place stresses and strains on the joints or pelvic floor. You are however advised to wait until after your 6 week postnatal check-up before returning to swimming, you can go a little earlier providing the discharge has stopped. It is important to be sure your body is sufficiently recovered and there is no risk of infection. Start off gently and build up the speed and distance gradually.

How often can I exercise?

At first you should see exercise as something to be integrated into your day as opposed to embarking on long and comprehensive exercise programmes. Caring for a new born baby can be quite physical in itself and, together with disturbed sleep, places quite strenuous demands on your body. At first being generally active, practising a few specific exercises and taking your baby out for walks will be sufficient. Look to gradually build up the length of your walks over the first 6 weeks, but remember – do not expect to do too much too soon.

The pelvic floor contractions and tummy tighteners prescribed in the postnatal programme 'one' are very gentle but extremely important exercises and should be practised as often as possible throughout the day. The other exercises within this very short programme, which should be practised at least once a day, can also easily be incorporated into daily activities. For example the squat exercise from postnatal programme 'one' can be practised whilst picking your baby up or putting him down.

After 6 weeks, and if you feel you can find the time and the energy to do more exercise, you can try the full exercise programme outlined in the postnatal programme 'two'. You need only do this programme every other day as your muscles need a day's rest between each exercise session to recover. However, the pelvic floor and tummy tighteners should become a part of your daily routine and you should continue to practise them as often as possible for the rest of your life!

When should I exercise in the day?

At first, it is unrealistic to think you can set yourself a regular time to exercise each day when you have to continually answer the demands of a newborn baby. However, after 6 weeks, when you may find your baby is beginning to fit into some sort of routine, aim to set aside some time – roughly the same each day – when you feel your baby will allow you a few minutes to yourself to exercise. It is important for you to find time to do something for yourself. You may feel the best time is when he is having a nap or you may prefer to include him in your exercise session, using it as a sort of play session at the same time. Suggestions are given within the exercises as to how you can exercise with your baby.

If you are breastfeeding it is always a good idea to exercise after a feed, as exercise can cause full breasts to leak.

How do I know I am doing enough?

For exercise to be effective you have to work hard enough to feel the effects of the exercise, nevertheless you should not work so hard as to end up feeling sore and exhausted. Check with the instructions for each exercise as to how much to aim for and what you should feel during each specific exercise.

The exercise programmes outlined concentrate on toning exercise – exercise that improves the shape, condition and firmness of muscles. The exercises will tire individual muscles more than leave you feeling out of breath. For toning exercise to be effective it has to make the muscles work a little bit more than they are comfortable with. You should therefore exercise a muscle until it aches a little, after a rest you could repeat the exercise until the muscle aches again. If you feel your muscles burning you have done too much. Rest them and move onto the next exercise.

When will I lose weight?

It is never advisable for mothers who are breast feeding to go on a diet although breast feeding is thought to enhance the weight loss process. By following a sensible approach to exercise and diet you will find your weight goes down quite naturally and your figure improves. Look to include plenty of walking into your weekly schedule as this effective form of aerobic exercise will contribute to sensible weight reduction. Mothers often find the last few pounds quite difficult to shift, in this case wait at least three months or until you have finished breastfeeding, then you can look to increase your exercise and perhaps reduce your intake if necessary. A flabby tummy months later is often due to a little excess fat and lack of muscle tone. Exercise and diet combined should solve the problem.

What makes a good exercise session?

Any comprehensive exercise session should start with a warm up and end with a cooldown. An adequate warm up consists of mobility exercises to loosen specific joints, some general rhythmic warming exercises to promote the circulation followed by some stretching exercises to promote an increased range of movement and relaxation within the muscles and joints. The body will then be warm and well prepared to work hard and safely in the main exercise session.

An adequate cooldown consists of stretching exercises to promote relaxation and suppleness within the muscles and joints. Since the muscles are warm at the end of the workout, it is an ideal time to stretch. Because of the effect of some hormones, stretches performed postnatally should generally be short and aim to promote relaxation rather than to increase suppleness. The cooldown should leave you feeling refreshed and relaxed, completing an invigorating, but not exhausting, exercise session.

The workout section of an exercise session will include toning or aerobic exercise – longer exercise sessions can include both. Toning exercise targets the muscles and consists of repetitions of a specific movement, curl-ups which work the abdominal muscles are an example of toning exercise. Toning exercise makes a major contribution to a firmer, more shapely, figure. Aerobic exercise works the heart and lungs and consists of rhythmical whole body movements to promote the circulation, raise the pulse and get you huffing and puffing a little. Brisk walking, jogging, cycling and swimming are all excellent aerobic activites. Aerobic exercise is very effective in burning up calories, making a major contribution to any weight loss programme.

Aim to incorporate some aerobic activity into your weekly schedule, for example walk at a brisk pace when taking your baby out for a breath of fresh air.

What you should know about the body
The effect of the hormone – Relaxin

In order for your body to accommodate the growing baby and facilitate childbirth, a hormone(relaxin) is released during pregnancy. Relaxin softens the fibrous tissue within the pelvis allowing it to expand slightly. Unfortunately the action of relaxin is not restricted to the pelvis – it affects all fibrous tissue in the body.

Relaxin and the joints
The effect of relaxin results in a slight softening of all the ligaments (the nuts and bolts of the joints) in the body, leading to a reduction in the stability of the joints. This can also lead to increased suppleness, an occurrence often noticed by women during pregnancy. Extra care is necessary when exercising to check that each exercise is performed correctly and carefully. This will ensure no excess stresses and strains are placed upon the joints which could increase the risk of injury. Check that you maintain correct body alignment and that you move with control throughout each exercise. The effect of relaxin gradually subsides following childbirth, but traces can be present for up to 5 months.

Relaxin and the muscles
Muscles are like a piece of elastic, they will stretch quite significantly and then easily return to their resting length. If, however, muscles are over stretched, as in the case of the abdominal muscles during pregnancy and the pelvic floor during childbirth, exercise is necessary to assist them to regain their tone.

The abdominal muscles
During pregnancy the abdominal muscles have to stretch to accommodate an increase in the waist measurement of about 20 inches and lengthen by about 8 inches. To allow for this increase around the waist, they often separate down the midline (above and below the tummy button along the line that can become more pigmented and brown during pregnancy) rather like a zip that splits open. It is important not to overstress these muscles once separation has occurred (in late pregnancy and the early postnatal period) so that it can repair itself satisfactorily afterwards. Postnatally these saggy muscles lack tone and as a result often fail to hold in the tummy to give you a flatter figure or support the spine in a way necessary to protect it from injury. The progression of abdominal exercises given in the exercise programmes will aid the repair of the separation and increase muscle tone. At first you will probably be alarmed at how saggy your tummy feels. Do not despair, practice your tummy exercises regularly – the bath is a great place to start as the buoyancy of the water assists you – and you will soon see progress being made.

Getting up from lying down

Because the abdominal muscles are weak and overstretched, it is important to avoid placing excess stress on them. When getting up from lying down, mothers are therefore advised to roll onto their side and use their arms to push themselves up to sitting rather than performing a straight forward sit up. The reverse applies when lying down.

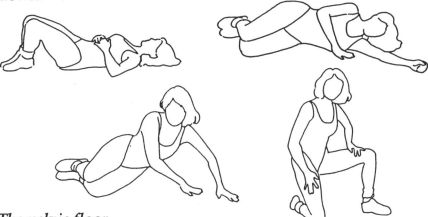

The pelvic floor

The pelvic floor is a sling of muscles that forms the floor of the pelvis and supports all the contents of the abdomen. Openings from the urethra, vagina and bowel all pass through this muscle layer which has to stretch like the neck of a poloneck jumper as the baby is born. The resulting lack of tone in this muscle often leads to a slight leak of urine on exertion (such as laughing or sneezing). This is a very common problem for mothers and is known as stress incontinence. Frequent practice of the pevlic floor exercise is necessary (and very effective) to avoid the problem persisting. Women should continue this exercise at frequent intervals during the day throughout their lives, as a well toned pelvic floor not only reduces the problems of stress incontinence, but also leads to an improved sex life. The pelvic floor contraction is detailed in the postnatal exercise programme 'one'.

Are you fit to exercise?

Providing you have not received any adverse instructions from your medical practitioners following childbirth, the postnatal programme 'one' will be totally safe for you to follow. After approximately 6 weeks – possibly 10 weeks if you had a caesarian – and following your postnatal check-up with your doctor, you can progress to the more demanding exercise programme (postnatal programme 'two')

providing you do not answer yes to any of the following questions.
• Do you get pains in your chest or has your doctor ever said you have heart disease, high blood pressure or any other cardiovascular problem?
• Do you suffer from painful or stiff joints which might be aggravated by exercise?
• Are you taking any medication at the moment?
• Do you have any other medical condition which may affect your ability to exercise?
If you have answered 'yes' to one or more questions, consult your doctor prior to embarking on the more comprehensive postnatal exercise programme 'two'.

Safety within the exercise session
• Check you have sufficient space that is free from obstacles in which to exercise.
• Never exercise in socks, bare feet is fine for these programmes.
• Wear a supporting bra and comfortable clothes that allow your body to breathe.
• Do not exercise following a meal, wait at least an hour for the food to be digested.
• Concentrate on the way you do each exercise – remember it is not only what you do, it's the way that you do it.
• If you are breastfeeding, to be comfortable, exercise following a feed.
• The exercise programmes together with the explanations detailed in this book are totally safe for you and will help you regain your figure quickly and effectively following childbirth. Be careful of following other exercise programmes as they may contain unsuitable exercises for example straight leg raises or straight leg situps.
• Exercise should never be painful, leave you feeling exhausted, or feeling stiff and sore the next day. If an exercise hurts or feels uncomfortable, relax from it then try again, checking your technique thoroughly. If it continues to be uncomfortable miss it out all together or seek further advice from an exercise professional. Many women experience severe discomfort in their pubis symphysis *(front of the pelvis)* during and after pregnancy. Some exercises, especially those that take the feet wide apart or involve twisting, can aggravate this discomfort. If this applies to you, miss out the exercise for a few weeks until you feel the discomfort disappears.

- Move with care and control throughout each exercise, never bounce or jerk.
- Don't expect to be able to do much at first. Be realistic and increase the amount of exercise you do gradually.

The exercise programmes

Before starting any exercise programme it is important that you check your posture. Good posture should be maintained throughout the day. During pregnancy, posture alters to accommodate the weight of the growing baby. Many women develop an increased curve in the lower back which places excess pressure on the lumbar spine. In the postnatal period, poor technique in lifting and carrying your baby plus heavy breasts which can cause you to stoop slightly (leading to round shoulders) can create further problems with posture. As a result it is important to work to regain body alignment and improve your posture at this time.

Cervical region *(upper back and neck)*

Good Posture

Neck extended, back of the head lifted tall, chin in and shoulders back and down.

Bad Posture

Drooping head, hunched and rounded shoulders, chin poking forwards.

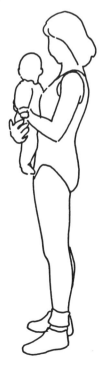 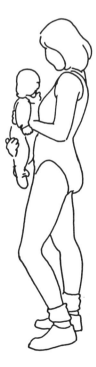

Thoracic region *(middle back)*
Good Posture
Ribs lifted, shoulder blades flat at the middle back and back straight, giving more room to breathe. The arms are working hard to support the baby.
Bad Posture
Shoulders rounded so that shoulder blades stick out, back bent forwards and lungs squashed.

Lumbar region *(lower back)*
Good Posture
Tummy flat and lower back lengthened as a result of pelvis being correctly tilted and weight distributed evenly over the legs with buttock muscles tight to stabilize the hips.
Bad Posture
Tummy stuck out and used to support the baby leading to an exaggerated curve *(lordosis)* in lower back; stress on the lower back due to the weight unevenly distributed over the legs.

Postnatal Exercise Programme 'One'

This programme is designed for you to begin as soon as possible following the birth of your baby.

As new exercises are described add them to those already practised on previous days so you build up to performing a series of safe, effective but easy and convenient exercises.

Aim to practise them as often as possible throughout the day – once you have mastered the exercise technique most can be done whilst holding your baby.

Days 1 & 2

1 Pelvic floor contraction
To retone the muscles of the pelvic floor

Sit up comfortably with your knees slightly apart and your feet flat on the floor. Think of drawing the pelvic floor muscles up inside, squeezing around the back, middle and front passages making sure you take it right to the front as if to hold back from having a wee. Hold this for a count of four then let go. Repeat 5 times an hour!

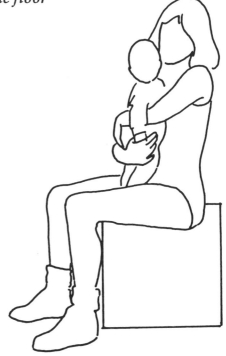

Feel that it is the muscles down below working – Check you are not holding your breath or tensing any other muscles at the same time – Once you have mastered the technique you can practise it standing, sitting or lying

2 Tummy tighteners – *An easy and accessible exercise to practise frequently for the abdominal muscles*
Sitting comfortably check that your feet are flat on the floor and your back is up straight. Without holding your breath, try to pull in your tummy so that the waistband of your skirt or trousers feels a little loose. Hold this for a count of 2, then relax. Repeat the exercise as often as possible and aim to increase the length of time you hold it. *Feel your tummy muscles working and aim to be able to hold them in until they ache a little – Check you do not hold your breath or tighten any other muscles at the same time*

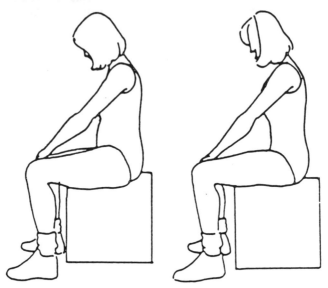

Days 3 & 4

3 Pelvic tilts – *To firm up the adominal muscles*
Lie on your back with your legs bent and your feet flat on the floor. Pulling in your tummy, tilt your pelvis up towards you so you see it dip in the middle and feel your lower back pressing into the floor. Relax and repeat 4 more times.
Feel your abdominal muscles working – You may find it helps to curl your buttocks slightly off the floor as well (check it's the abdominals working, not your leg muscles) – Ensure you are not holding your breath

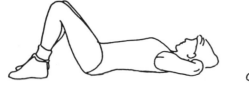
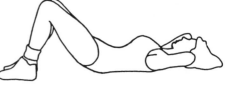

4 Alternate heel raises – *To promote circulation to the feet and ankles*

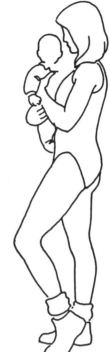

Standing tall with your feet hip width apart, raise one heel pressing the ball of the foot into the ground. Change feet raising the heel of the other foot off the ground. Increase the speed of the movement to resemble walking through the feet on the spot. Continue for about 1 minute.

Feel the calf muscles working – Check your posture and that your hips stay level to reduce the stress on the pelvis – Keep the weight over the big toe, press the ball of the foot into the floor

Days 5 & 6

5 Kneeling hips hitches – *To tone the abdominal obliques (the muscles around the waist)*

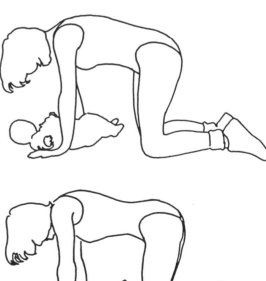

Adopt a position on all fours with your knees directly beneath your hips and your hands directly beneath your shoulders. Keep your abdominals pulled in tightly to keep your back flat. Slowly and with control, sway your bottom from side to side, squeezing your waist muscles and drawing your hip up towards your ribs on one side and then the other. Do this 16 times in total.

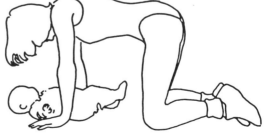

Feel the muscles in your waist tighten – Check you do not allow your back to dip – Keep your arms straight and your shoulders still

6 Squats – *To strengthen the thigh muscles and develop good technique for lifting and carrying*

Stand over your baby with your feet apart, one foot facing forwards and the other pointing very slightly out. Bending very slightly forwards at the hips and pulling your tummy in to support your back, bend your knees, checking they follow the line of your feet until your hips are level with your knees. Reach your arms down to your baby and pick him up drawing him in close to you before straightening you legs. Give your muscles a rest before trying this exercise again.

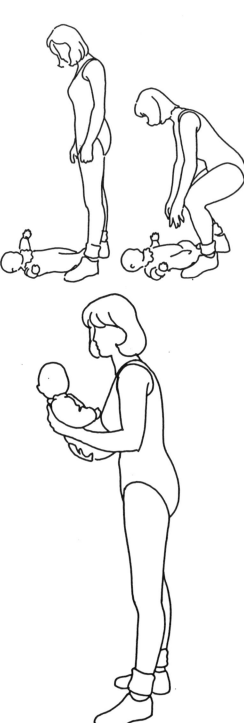

Feel your thigh muscles working – You may also feel a slight stretch at the top of your legs around the inner thighs – Check that your shoulders stay higher than your hips and your hips stay higher than your knees – Keep the heel of your front foot down, the heel of the back foot may rise up slightly – Tighten your pelvic floor as you pick up the baby – Think of pushing your knees out as you bend them so they stay in line with your feet – Hold baby in close to you supporting his head and keep your back up straight as you stand up.

Day 7
7 Easy curl-ups – *To strengthen the abdominal muscles*

Lie on your back, both legs bent, feet flat on the floor and your head resting on a pillow to lift it slightly. Place one hand behind your head for support and the other on your thigh. Pulling in your abdominals to flatten your tummy and looking towards your knees, lift your head slightly off the pillow sliding your hand a little way up your thigh. Relax and repeat the exercise up to 4 more times.

Feel your abdominal muscles working – Rest your head in your hand for support and to ease the comfort of your neck – It is a good idea to practice this exercise whilst in the bath as the buoyancy of the water assists the curl-up and it is easy to check that you are doing it correctly – Check your tummy stays flat throughout the curl-up. If it bunches up or domes avoid this exercise for a few more days and continue with the tummy tighteners and pelvic tilts. The doming is caused by the weakness of the abdominal muscles and the separation of the two sides of the long muscle down the front. You can test for separation by; placing two fingers crosswise above or below the naval and pressing them into this centre line then raise your head and you will find the two sides clip/squeeze your fingers if separation is present.

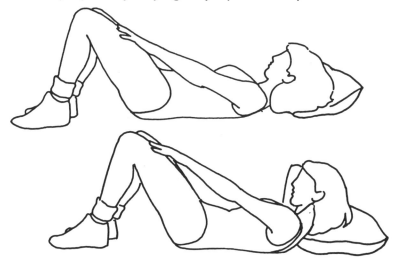

– You can progress this exercise by placing both hands lightly behind your head and keeping your elbows out sideways as you curl up

Continue to practice all these exercises daily for the next few weeks. As you feel your abdominal muscles strengthening you can aim to curl-up a little higher (on condition that your muscles do not dome) in the easy curl-up exercise.

Postnatal Exercise Programme 'Two'

Following your postnatal checkup, aim to follow this 12 minute programme every other day.

Take time at first to learn the exercises correctly then work to establish a rhythm that suits you.

The more effort you put into the exercises the more effective they will be, concentrate on good technique, moving with control and following a full range of movement within each exercise.

Don't forget to practise the pelvic floor exercise. Do 4 before you start.

WARM UP EXERCISES

1 Knee bends and alternate arm circles – *To promote the circulation and warm you up*

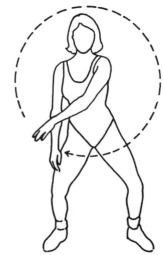

Stand with your feet just over shoulder width apart and your toes pointing slightly out. Keeping your heels pressed into the ground, your tummy in tight and your back upright, slowly bend and straighten your legs, at the same time, circling one arm across your body, up over your head and out to the side. Repeat the exercise 7 more times circling alternate arms.

Put lots of effort into the exercise and feel the movement loosening the shoulders – You should begin to feel warm after a few repetitions

Repeat this exercise after each of the following 6 mobility exercises.

2 Shoulder circles – *To loosen the shoulders and upper back*
Stand with your feet shoulder width apart and your arms hanging loosely by your sides. Roll your shoulders in as large a circle as possible taking them forwards, up, squeezing them back and dropping them down. Repeat 7 more times.
Feel the muscles of the chest and top of the back working and relaxing – Make the movement as large as possible – Keep your tummy pulled in tightly to keep your lower back still.

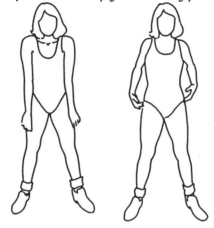

Repeat knee bends and arm circles

3 Reaches – *To reduce stiffness in the sides of the body and warm the muscles*
Stand with your feet slightly wider than hip width apart and tummy held in tightly to support your back. Extend one arm above your head and reach for the ceiling. Drop the shoulder on the other side. Relax and repeat the exercise 7 more times using alternate arms.
Look up towards your hand and feel a full extension down your side – Do not twist or bend to the side

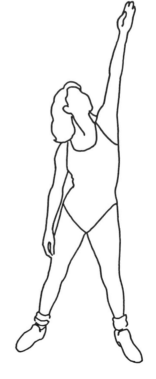

Repeat knee bends and arm circles

4 Hip wiggles – *To mobilise the lower back*

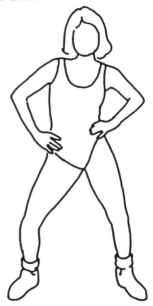

Stand with your feet slightly wider than shoulder width apart, your knees slightly bent and your hands on your hips. Keeping your weight evenly distributed between your feet, tighten your waist muscles and draw your hips up towards your ribs on one side. Relax and repeat to the other side. Repeat the exercise alternating sides until you have done it 8 times on both sides.

Feel your waist muscles working – Aim to keep your knees and shoulders still
Repeat knee bends and arm circles

5 Waist twists – *To mobilise the spine*

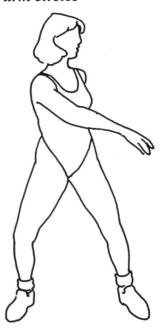

Stand with good posture, your feet slightly wider than shoulder width apart. Keeping your hips still and facing the front, slowly twist your head, shoulders and arms round to one side, reaching round with your arms as far as possible. Return to the start position and repeat the exercise alternating sides until you have done 6 twists in total.

Feel the movement stretching and working the muscles in the trunk –
Squeeze your buttocks to help you keep your hips still
Repeat knee bends and arm circles

6 Ankle circles – *To reduce any stiffness in the ankle joints*

Standing on one leg rest the toes of the other foot on the floor slightly to the side. Keeping your hips still, circle the ankle clockwise, making the movement as large as possible. Do 4 full circles then repeat with the other foot.

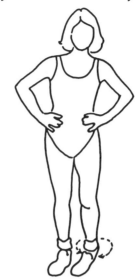

Feel the movement mobilising the ankle joint – Keep the foot in light contact with the floor

Repeat knee bends and arm circles

7 Knee lifts – *To mobilise the hip joints and promote the circulation*
Stand tall with good posture, your feet hip width apart and your arms extended out to the sides at shoulder height. Lifting one knee up towards your chest, bring your arms forwards to end up in front of you at shoulder height. Return to the start position and repeat the exercise using alternate legs until you have done it 16 times in total. *Hold your abdominal muscles in tightly to stabilise your back – Keep the supporting leg straight as you lift the other knee*

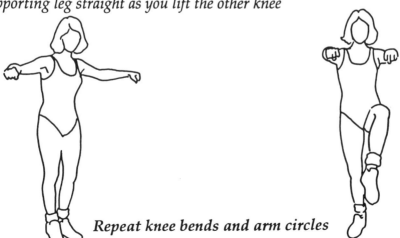

Repeat knee bends and arm circles

8 Shoulder stretch – *To relax the muscles of the trunk and shoulders*

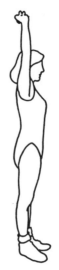

Stand with good posture, your feet hip width apart and your toes pointing forwards. Clasp your hands together and, keeping your tummy held in tightly, pull in your abdominals and extend your arms above your head. Reach them up and back until you feel the stretch around your shoulders and your middle. Hold for a slow count of 4, relax and repeat.

Check you do not hold your breath – Try to take your arms behind your ears without allowing your back to arch

9 Side stretch – *To stretch the muscles around the waist (obliques)*

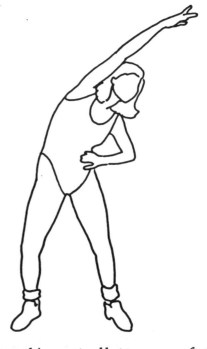

Stand with your feet a little wider than shoulder-width apart, knees bent and one hand resting on one hip for support. Reach up to the ceiling with the other arm. Tilt your pelvis to straighten your lower back then, breathing out, bend sideways, over towards the supporting arm. Reach up and over your head with the extended arm until you feel a stretch down the opposite side of your body. Hold for a slow count of 4, relax and repeat for the other side. Repeat on both sides.

Don't lean forwards or backwards – Keep your hips centred between your feet

10 Inner thigh stretch – *To stretch the muscles along the inner thigh (adductors)*

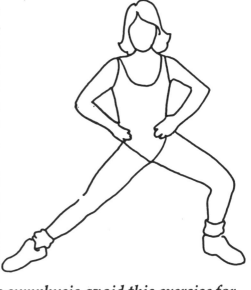

Stand with your feet wide apart and your toes pointing slightly out. Bend one knee, keeping your weight evenly distributed between your feet, slide the other leg away sideways, keeping it straight, until you feel a stretch in your inner thigh. Hold for a slow count of 4, repeat to the other side. Repeat the stretch to both sides.
Keep both hips facing forwards and the feet flat on the floor – If you don't feel a stretch, check your feet are wide enough apart and your weight is evenly distributed between them, bend your supporting leg a little more.
If you feel discomfort in the pubis symphysis avoid this exercise for a few weeks

11 Quad stretch – *To stretch the muscles along the front of the thigh (quadriceps)*

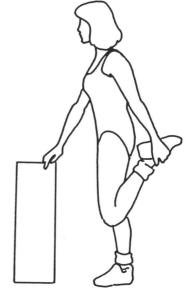

Stand on one leg with knee slightly bent and hold onto a chair for support. Tuck your bottom under and tighten your abdominals to stabilise your back, bring the heel of the other leg back and up towards the buttocks. Hold your ankle and lift your foot to bring the heel in towards your buttocks until you feel a stretch down the front of your thigh. Hold for a slow count of 4, relax and repeat with the other leg. Repeat the stretch for both legs.
Hold the abdominals in tightly to stop the back arching – Keep your thighs parallel (your knees do not have to be together) – If you cannot reach your ankle, loop a towel around it and pull on that

12 Hamstring stretch – *To stretch the muscles along the back of the thigh (hamstrings)*

Stand with feet hip width apart, one foot slightly in front of the other. Place your hands on the thigh of the back leg for support. Sticking your bottom backwards and pulling your shoulders back to keep your back straight, bend forwards from the hips until you feel a stretch in the back of your front leg. Hold for a slow count of 4, relax and repeat for the other leg. Repeat for both legs.

Check you bend forwards from the hips and keep your back as straight as possible – Do not expect to bend very far

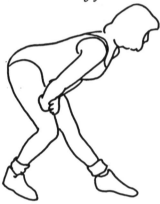

13 Calf stretch – *To stretch the muscles around the back of the upper calf (gastrocnemius). Good for cramp*

Stand with one foot in front and one foot behind, pointing forwards, hip-width apart. Keep the back leg straight and the heel pressed into the floor, bend your front leg until you feel a stretch in the back of the rear leg just below the knee. Hold for a slow count of 4, change legs and repeat. Repeat the stretch for both calfs.

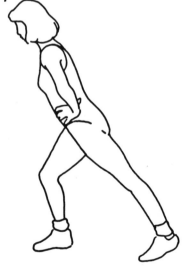

If you find it difficult to balance, check the feet are not one behind the other – If you feel uncomfortable or cannot feel a stretch, move the back leg back slightly, check it is straight and the heel pressed into the floor

14 Lower calf stretch – *To stretch the lower calf muscles (soleus)*
Stand in the front and back astride position as for the previous calf
stretch. Tightening your abdominals to keep your lower back straight
and keeping your heels pressed into the ground, bend your knees
until you feel a stretch down the back of the calf towards the ankle.
Hold for a slow count of 4, change legs and repeat. Repeat the stretch
for both legs.
*Check that your feet both face forwards and your knees point in the same
direction as your feet – Tighten your buttock muscles to support the hips –
If you have trouble balancing, check that your feet are wide enough apart*

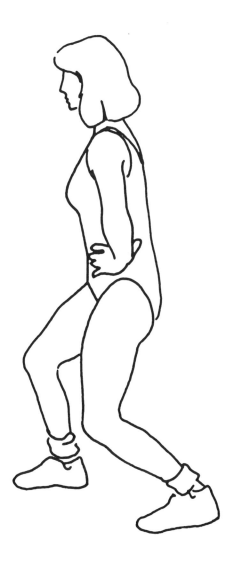

WORKOUT EXERCISES

1 Armwork –*To tone up the muscles in the front and back of the arms (biceps and triceps), reducing flab*
Stand with your feet hip width apart and your elbows tucked into your waist. Keeping your elbows tucked in, bend your arms bringing your hands up towards your shoulders. Extend your arms again then, keeping them straight, slowly lift them backwards as far as possible. Repeat the exercise until you have done it 8 times.
For more effect hold something weighing a pound or two – Keep your tummy tight and back still – Try to lift the arms that little bit higher at the back

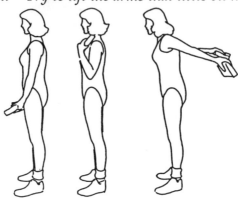

2 Elbow squeezes – *To tone the chest muscles (pectorals) and contribute towards a better figure*
Stand with your feet hip width apart and your arms out sideways and bent, elbows at shoulder height, fists towards the ceiling. Keeping your arms bent, elbow high and your fist towards the ceiling, bring your arms in aiming to squeeze your elbows together. Return to the start position and repeat until you have done 8in total.
Feel the chest muscles working – Keep your tummy pulled in tightly to stabilise your back – If your breasts are full or sore miss out this exercise

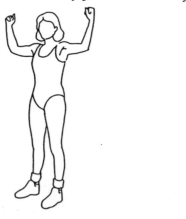
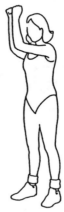

3 Knee bends – *To strengthen and tone the muscles along the front of the thigh (quadriceps). Important for many day-to-day tasks as well as appearance*

Stand with your feet hip width apart, toes pointing forwards and abdominals pulled in tightly. Leaning very slightly forwards from the hips and keeping your heels on the floor, bend your knees as far as possible without letting your hips drop below your knees. Return to start position. Repeat this exercise until you have done it 8 times. *Feel your thigh muscles working – Check that your knees bend in line with your feet*

4 Box pressups – *To tone the muscles of the arms and chest*

Adopt a position on all fours with your hands directly under your shoulders and your knees directly under your hips. *(Lie your baby on the floor beneath you for this).* Pulling in your abdominals, bend your elbows lowering your face towards your baby. Push up slowly to return to the start position. Aim to do 8.

– Feel the muscles in your chest and arms working – Do not allow your back to dip – Breathe out as you push up – To progress this exercise, lay baby so that his head is a little in front of your hands. Before bending your arms shift your hips and shoulders forwards a little to place slightly more weight on your hands. Keeping the weight forwards bend your arms

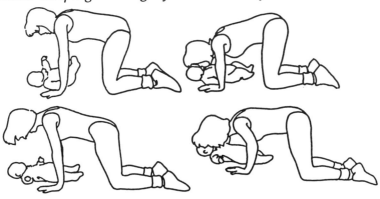

5 Kneeling rear leg raises – *To tone the buttock muscles (gluteals) leading to a more shapely behind!*
Adopt an all fours position as for pressups. Extend one leg out behind keeping your toes lightly in touch with the floor. *(Your baby can lie on the floor between your arms)*. Keeping your abdominals tight to stabilise your back and your hips square to the floor, slowly raise the straight leg until it is horizontal to the floor. Relax and repeat 7 times. Change legs and repeat 8 times on the other leg.
Feel your buttock muscles working – Check you do not allow your back to dip or twist

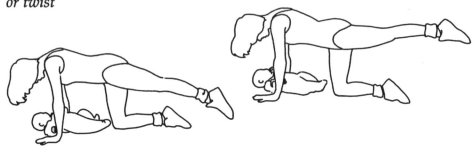

6 Kneeling rear leg curls –*To tone the muscles at the back of the thigh (hamstrings) for a more shapely behind!*
Adopt a position on all fours, extend one leg out behind you as before. Raise this leg until it is level with your back and horizontal to the floor. Keeping the back flat, hips square to the floor and knee still, bend the leg bringing the heel in towards your buttock. Extend the leg again and repeat 7 times. Change legs and repeat the exercise 8 times for the other leg.
– Feel the muscles at the back of the thigh working – Concentrate on squeezing the heel in towards the buttocks to make the exercise more effective

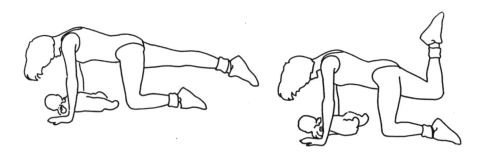

ABDOMINAL EXERCISES

Do not attempt to do all of the following 4 exercises the first time you try this programme. Add one new exercise each week over the next four.

1 Curl-ups – *To strengthen the abdominal muscles for a flat tum and provide good stability to the lumbar spine*
Lie on your back with your knees bent and your feet flat on the floor. You can rest your baby on your thighs or sit him on your hips if you wish. Ensure that you hold on to him tightly with both hands. Pulling in your abdominals to tighten and flatten your tummy, curl your head and shoulders a little way of the floor then lower yourself gently back to the start position. Build up to 8 repetitions in one go.
Feel your abdominal muscles working – Check that your tummy does not dome – Breathe out as you curl up – You can progress by aiming to curl up a little higher, and eventually high enough to give your baby a kiss!

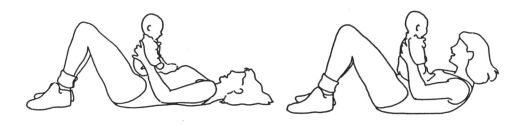

You can also make the exercise harder by sitting the baby higher up your body, as he gets heavier the exercise will get harder!

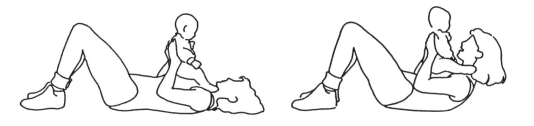

2 Twisting curl-ups – *To provide conditioning for the abdominals with an emphasis on the obliques and contribute towards a flat tum*
Only progress to this exercise if your abdominals have repaired from separation (see page 59)
Lie on your back with knees bent and head gently resting in your fingertips. Keeping your elbows back and your abdominals held in firmly to keep your tummy flat, curl up with a twist bringing one knee in to meet the opposite elbow. Return to the start position and repeat on the other side. Aim to do 8 repetitions in one go.
Feel your abdominals working – Only curl up as far, or as many times, as you can with your tummy staying flat – Check you do not pull on your head with your hands or hold your breath

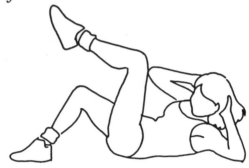

3 Lying side bends – *To tone the waist muscles (abdominal obliques) and contribute to a flat tum*
Only progress to this exercise if your abdominals have repaired from separation (see page 59)
Lie on your back with both knees bent and your feet flat on the ground. Rest your head in your finger tips. Curl your head and shoulders very slightly off the ground then bend to one side reaching round to touch your heel one side with your fingertips. Return to the start position and repeat to the other side. Aim to be able to do 8 repetitions in one go.
Feel your tummy muscles working especially around your waist – Only do as many as you can do correctly with your tummy flat – Breathe out as you reach round to your heel

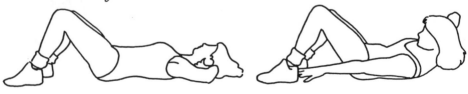

4 Lying side leg raises – *To strengthen and tone the muscles of the hips and the outside of the thigh (abductors).*

Lie on your side with the underneath leg bent (for balance) the top leg straight (in line with your body) and your head resting in your hand as illustrated. Making sure your hips and tummy face forward and, keeping the hips completely still, slowly raise and lower your straight leg. Do this 8 times.

Feel the muscles down the outside of hip and thigh working – To make the exercise harder, lift your leg as high as you can without twisting the hips

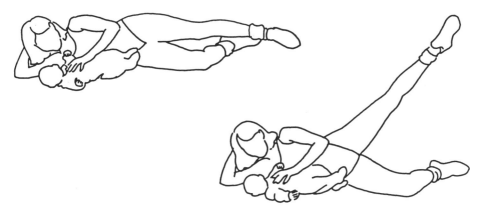

5 Sitting inner thigh squeezes – *To tone the inner thigh muscles (adductors), an area that can often become flabby following childbirth*

Sit up straight with good posture, on the floor or a chair, and a small cushion between your knees. Breathing out and relaxing all the other muscles in the body, squeeze your knees together and hold for a slow count of 2. Relax. Do this 8 times.

Feel your inner thigh muscles working

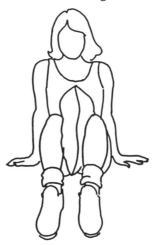

COOLDOWN STRETCHES
Begin with a pelvic floor contraction.
1 Sitting hamstring stretch – *To relax the muscles at the back of the thigh (hamstrings) promoting a feeling of relaxation*
Sit on the floor with one leg straight out in front of you and the other leg bent slightly to the side. Pulling in your tummy muscles and, trying to keep your back straight, slowly bend forwards from the hips over the straight leg until you feel a stretch down the back of this leg. Hold the stretch for a slow count of 8 then relax and repeat on the other leg.
If you feel a pull in your back adjust the position of the bent leg – Concentrate on relaxing into the stretch, bending from the hips not the upper back – Do not bounce

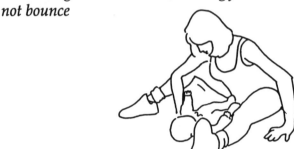

2 Side lying quad stretch – *To relax the muscles down the front of the thigh (quadriceps). These muscles can become quite tight and as a result contribute to poor posture*
Lie on your side with the underneath leg bent for balance, and your head resting in your hand as illustrated. Keeping your back firm and straight, bend the top leg and clasp your ankle with your spare hand. Gently ease the heel in towards your buttocks and take the knee back until you feel a stretch down the front of the thigh. Hold the stretch for a slow count of 8, relax and repeat on the other leg.
Try to relax in to the stretch – Check your back does not arch

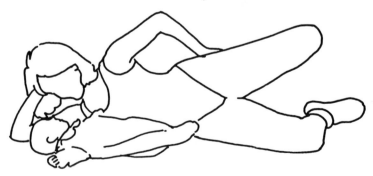

3 Taylor stretch – *To stretch the inner thigh muscles (adductors). Releasing tension in these muscles is important to facilitate correct technique when picking baby up off the floor*
Sit on the floor with your legs bent, the soles of your feet together and your feet as close to your body as possible. You can rest back on your hands. Allow your knees to flop apart and the weight on your legs to bring about the stretch in the inner thigh. Hold the stretch for a slow count of 8.
Try to relax the muscles, do not bounce or jerk – You can assist the stretch by holding your ankles and gently pressing your knees out with your elbows

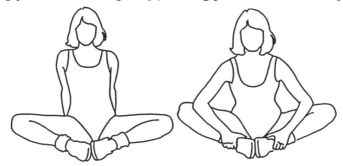

4 Sitting buttock stretch – *To stretch the buttock muscles (gluteals). Important for good lifting and bending technique*
In a sitting position, leaning back on your hands for support, bend one leg placing the foot flat on the floor a little way away from you. Bend your arms slightly to give yourself room between your chest and the thigh of the bent leg. Bend the spare leg resting the ankle, not the foot, across the knee of the other leg. Using your arms, straighten your back and think of folding at the hip joint, move your ribs up towards your thighs until you feel a stretch in the buttocks on one side. Repeat reversing the position of the legs.
Keep the knee of the side being stretched as far away from you as possible – Think of lifting up from the lower back

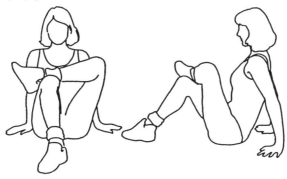

5 Kneeling shoulder stretch – *To stretch the muscles around the shoulder joints*

Adopt a kneeling position with your buttocks on your heels, your arms extended in front of you, your hands on the floor, thumbs close together and chest resting on thighs. Keeping your chest low, slide your hands and hips forward, raising your buttocks up off your heels until your hips are directly above your knees. Keeping hips high and arms out straight, push your chest down towards your knees until you feel a stretch in your shoulders. Hold the stretch for a slow count of 8.

Think of a weight pressing down on your shoulder blades – Hold your tummy in firmly to ensure your back does not arch – Check your hips are not in front of, or behind, your knees, you should feel comfortable and balanced

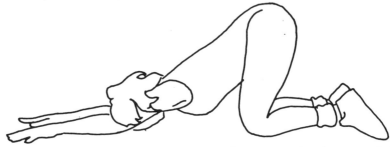

6 Sitting chest stretch – *To stretch the chest muscles (pectorals) and relieve any tension caused by heavy breasts*

Sit up tall on the floor with your knees bent and your feet flat on the floor. Place your fingertips lightly on the floor behind you. Squeezing your shoulder blades together and thinking of expanding your chest, lift your chest so that it move up towards the ceiling. Look up as well until you feel a stretch across the front. Hold the stretch for a slow count of 4, rest and then repeat.

Rest on your fingertips for support –

Don't allow the head to fall backwards

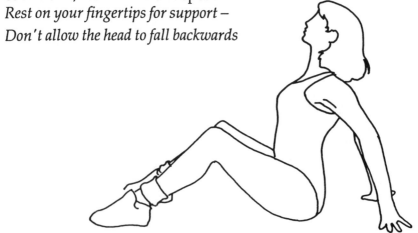

When can I return to exercise classes?

Exercise classes can be safely returned to following your 6 week postnatal check-up with your doctor. Any return however must be gradual and you should not look to start exercising at the level you achieved before your pregnancy. Progress will occur at quite a rate but listen to your body and do not overdo it.

If possible, start with a specific postnatal exercise class for the first few weeks following your 6 week check-up and progress to a beginner class before returning to your more advanced and intense workout. Check your technique carefully to minimise stresses on the lower back or pelvis and only perform abdominal exercises to a degree where you can maintain a flat stomach. If doming occurs the muscles have either become fatigued or the exercise is too demanding. In these instances stop the excercises or seek alternatives.

Exercise classes often include a comprehensive stretch section in the cool-down during which *'developmental stretching'* is employed to encourage an increase in flexibility. Because of the effect of relaxin, extra care should be taken when performing stretching exercises and women are not encouraged to perform developmental stretching for at least 5 months after childbirth. Keep the stretches short and stretch to promote relaxation rather than stretching to improve flexibility.

Avoid impact work in an aerobics class until you feel your pelvic floor has regained its full tone and elasticity. It is important not to stress an already weakened muscle. If you suffer from stress incontinence, work even harder at your pelvic floor exercises. Impact work also places a high degree of stress on your joints and muscles. Remember, traces of the hormone relaxin can be present for some time and this will affect the ability of your joints to sustain these extra stresses.

Summary

The changes that took place in your body during your pregnancy will affect you for some time following the birth of your baby. Whilst it is not true that you are 'never the same again', recovery should be gradual. Attempts to expect or do too much too soon can lead to problems while the body is still affected by hormones and learning to cope with the added demands of a new baby. It is never too late to start exercise following childbirth but you should always commence very gently and then progress gradually at a rate that is comfortable to you. Understanding the changes that have occurred during pregnancy and how they affect you postnatally will also help. Listen to your body and be confident that this guide will help you regain your figure with ease and interest.

Follow these guidelines to be as safe as posssible in your efforts to regain your figure:–

• *Follow a gentle programme of abdominal muscles exercises. Do not strain them or perform straight leg raises/situps*

• *Practise pelvic floor contractions regularly*

• *Keep a little time each day for the 12 minute toning programme for improved muscle tone*

• *Stand and carry your baby with good posture*

• *Do not diet and exercise excessively*

• *Try some gentle aerobic exericise daily (walking)*

• *If breastfeeding, exercise following a feed*

Above all, remember to listen to your body, take it gradually but be determined to persevere. A little regular exercise will help you to achieve a firm and shapely body.

HIP AND THIGH EXERCISES

and

FLATTEN YOUR STOMACH

by

Becca Thompson

Introduction

It is important to stand and exercise with good posture. Before starting any exercises, ensure you are in the good posture position. Stand with feet shoulder width apart and slightly turned out.

These exercises are both simple and effective, so you won't need a degree to understand them. They are not a total exercise programme. To achieve a full degree of fitness the exercises illustrated should be combined with total body exercises and aerobic exercise for the heart and lungs such as dance, swimming, cycling etc.

You should aim to carry out some form of exercise programme 3 times a week. However if you do these exercises on a regular basis you will see and feel improvement in the shape and tone of your body.

Are you fit enough?

Exercising is the key to a fit and healthy body; however it does not suit everyone and some can be adversely effected by exercise.

Ask yourself some simple questions before trying these exercises. If the answer is *'yes'* to one or more of the questions below consult your doctor. If you answered *'no'* to the questions, then you are ready to start. So have fun and think of the benefits!

Questions

- Has your doctor ever advised you that you have heart trouble or is there a history of heart disease in your family?
- Do you often have pains in your heart or chest?
- Do you have dizzy spells, headaches or suffer from fainting?
- Do you have problems with any joints especially those that have been aggravated by exercise?
- Are you presently taking any medication?
- Do you have any other medical condition which makes you think you may not be able to exercise? If you are at all unsure check with your doctor first.

Safety

It is imperative to prepare body and mind for strenuous exercise. Listed are 'warm up' exercises to stretch and prepare the muscles; warm muscles work more effectively & prevent injury. It is essential to allow the heart and lungs time to gradually accustomise to strenuous activity.

After exercising the body must be given time to recover, and the 'cooldown' section suggests stretches for the specific muscle groups used.

So always remember 'Warm up' and 'Cooldown'.

Never exercise on a full stomach. Don't eat or drink *(except water)* when exercising. Having started, maintain continuity and having completed the warm up go straight to the toning exercises. Do not take a tea break in between. Always *stop* if any exercise or stretch hurts. Recheck your exercise position against the diagram or try an alternative exercise working the same muscle group. If you still feel uncomfortable then please *stop*. Don't force stretch positions, never bounce or hold a stretch for too long. If you are unused to regular exercise they may take a while to become comfortable so only hold for 6-8 seconds and build up gradually. It is essential not to overdo things in the beginning. The best results will be achieved by a slow, gradual build up of exercises carried out on a regular basis.

Posture check

Think about your posture and your body alignment. This applies in everyday life as well as during exercise! Stand tall with your feet 'hip' width apart & tilt the pelvis forward slightly pulling the stomach in and tucking your bottom under. Raise the shoulders up, push them back and drop them down, keeping them relaxed. The back should be straight and the head held high. Remember, keep the knees slightly bent, *never* lock out the joints. We refer to this position throughout the book, so make sure you master it.

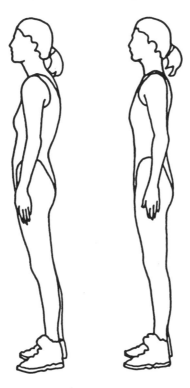

Warm up

You must prepare the body and mind. By trying a few simple exercises you can prevent injury and soreness in the muscles and joints. 'MOBILITY' exercises are included to 'loosen up' the joints; by performing smooth movements to stimulate fluid in the joint, which allows for improved movement and prevents injury.

The warm up also includes 'PULSE RAISING' exercises such as swing steps and knee lifts. These gradually increase the body temperature and allow time for the extra blood supply to reach the muscles in the more strenuous toning exercises. This reduces the risk of muscle soreness. Before starting ensure you have read and answered 'Are You Fit Enough?'. Also make sure you have enough room to exercise comfortably preferably on a carpeted area, or using a towel or mat as a base, perhaps play some cheerful music to help you exercise. It is also important to wear comfortable clothing. You don't have to wear aerobic kit, just clothes that won't restrict your movements whilst exercising. The warm up exercises are designed to help you attain the maximum benefits – safely – from your toning exercises and therefore help you achieve the best results overall.

Toning

Having completed your warm up you are now ready to do the toning exercises. These are designed to work specific areas and will increase the strength and endurance of the muscles and improve their shape and tone.

This is achieved by positive overload. This simply means when the muscle is put in a situation where it must work against a greater level of stress than it is used to, when you reach muscle fatigue – *not pain.* This is done by increasing the intensity and resistance of an exercise. It is very important to alternate these exercises between the different muscle groups and not overwork and tire one muscle group.

Always choose A or B of an exercise, do not do both. Don't, on the other hand, do 4 exercises all for the same muscle group as you will undoubtedly feel discomfort in this area.

Always build up the intensity gradually on each exercise – try to exhale as you exert the effort and inhale as you relax on all the exercises. Each diagram shows a shaded area which indicates where you should feel the benefit of the exercise or stretch. Obviously we are all different and it may vary slightly. If you do not feel the exercise in the same area as shown in the diagram re-check and possibly re-adjust your exercise position as just a slight realignment of the knee or toe can adjust the muscle groups you are aiming to work. Above all in this section remember to do these exercises at your own pace, take a rest between sets if you want to and always stop if it hurts.   Try to enjoy yourself whilst exercising and think of the improvements you are making.

Cooldown

After your toning exercises it is important to do some cooldown stretches which prevent stiffness and soreness in the joints and muscles. This time also allows the body to return to its pre-exercising state both mentally and physically.   During the toning exercises the muscles become shortened yet with some simple stretches the muscles will return to their pre-exercising length.   As the muscles are warmer after exercising you can hold the stretches for a little longer, between 10-20 seconds.   This will help to increase their range and flexibility.

It is important to remember stretching is very individual and you should only stretch as far as is comfortable for you – *listen to your body*. You should hold the stretch and be aware of a mild tension as the muscle lengthens but it should not be painful. *Never bounce* or *force* a stretch position as this will evoke a 'stretch reflex' which means the muscle automatically contracts to protect itself from being overstretched.   If this occurs the muscle is unable to relax and lengthen properly. For the best results be patient and do the stretches regularly. You should always try to relax and breathe normally throughout this section and at the end you should feel relaxed and refreshed.

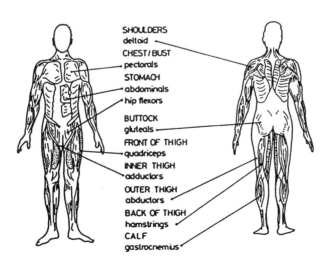

SHOULDERS
deltoid
CHEST / BUST
pectorals
STOMACH
abdominals
hip flexors

BUTTOCK
gluteals
FRONT OF THIGH
quadriceps
INNER THIGH
adductors
OUTER THIGH
abductors
BACK OF THIGH
hamstrings
CALF
gastrocnemius

WARM UP EXERCISES

1 Shoulder rolls

Assume correct posture check position. Bring the shoulders forward, lift them up and rotate them backwards. Keep the movement slow and controlled. This promotes feeling of loosening up the shoulder joints. Repeat this 4 times then rotate the shoulders forwards 4 times.

2 Head side to side

Assume correct posture check position. With the shoulders down and relaxed, look to your right shoulder, (not over the shoulder) just enough that your chin is level with your shoulder. Then look to the left shoulder. Repeat 4 times each side. Always face forwards and then turn the head, this gently eases out the neck. *Never* swing from side to side.

3 Side bends

Assume correct posture check position. With the right arm outstretched reach away from the side of the body, simultaneously lifting the elbow of the left arm to shoulder height, the upper body reaches to the right hand side creating a stretch all along the left hand side of the body. Keep the hips and shoulders facing forwards, slowly return to the centre before repeating. *Don't swing*. Repeat 4 times each side.

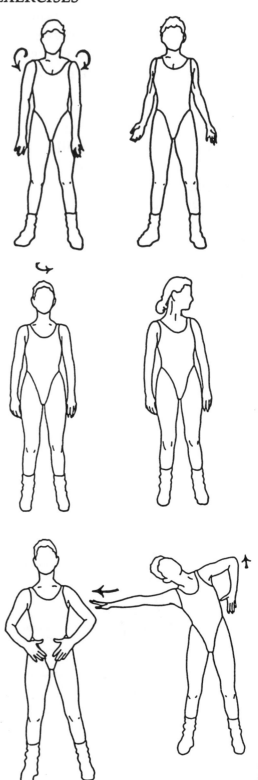

4 Hip circles

Assume correct posture check position. Circle the hips keeping the stomach pulled in. Be careful not to arch the back. Keep the movement slow and controlled. This creates a feeling of 'loosening up' in the lower back. Keep the knees soft and upper body still. Repeat 4 circles in each direction.

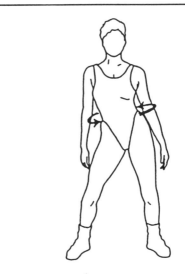

5 Knee bends

Take the feet a good distance apart with the feet turned out slightly at 45°. Keeping the stomach pulled in, the back straight and pelvis tilted forwards bend and straighten the legs. Be sure not to lock out the knees as you come up. The knees go out over the toes not facing forwards. Do not bend to far as this is only a warm up exercise. Repeat 8 times. Then repeat 8 times adding the arms reaching down and pulling the elbows upto chest height.

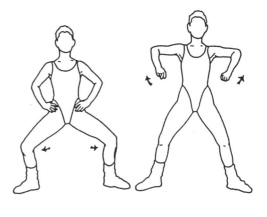

6 Marches

Assume the correct posture check position. Then bring the feet together and march on the spot. Do not stamp the feet. Keep the back straight and the stomach pulled in. Stand tall. Swing the arms and lift the knees a little higher to add some effort. Repeat 16 times.

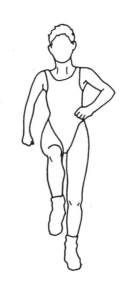

7 Heels in front

Assume correct posture check position. Push one heel out in front, flexing the foot. Bend the supporting leg at the same time, alternate on each leg. Repeat 8 times. Then repeat 8 times adding bicep curls with the arms. Bend the elbows and pull the fists in towards the chest. Alternate 8 times without arms, 8 times with.

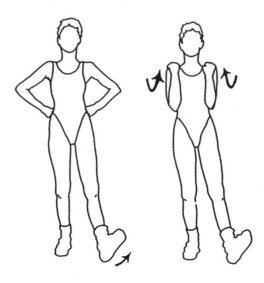

8 Knees lift

Assume correct posture check position. Lift alternate knees to the chest keeping your back straight, don't slouch over as you lift the knee. Keep the supporting leg soft don't lock out the knee. Repeat 8 times. Repeat 8 times adding the arm movements. Reach forward with both arms at shoulder height. Now repeat exercises 7 and 8. If you find it confusing using the arm and leg movements leave out the arm movements until you become more familiar with the exercises.

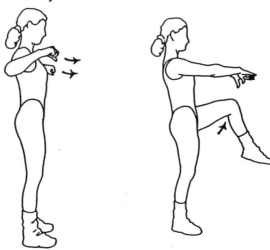

9 Swing step

Take the feet wide apart and step from one foot to the other. Bend the knees through the middle as you transfer your weight. At the same time swing the arms at shoulder height. The more effort you put into this exercise by taking larger steps and bending more in the middle the warmer you become. Repeat for 8 swings.

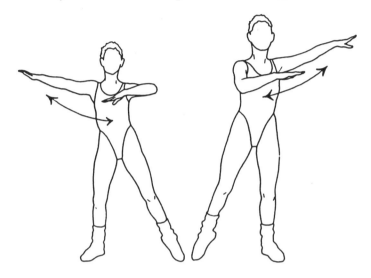

10 Swing step & heel raise

Repeat as above, at the same time lift alternate heels in towards the bottom. Make sure your supporting leg is always bent. Don't lock out the knees. Repeat 8 times. Now repeat exercises 9 and 10.

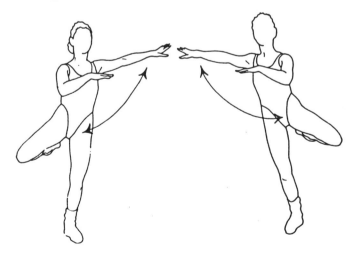

You should now feel warmer and ready to stretch, if however you do not repeat exercises 7 to 10

WARM UP STRETCHES

11 Front thigh   *Quadricep*

Assume the correct posture check position. Bend the left supporting leg slightly and draw the opposite heel in towards the bottom holding the foot near the ankle (not curling the toes). Keep the hips square and pushed forward and the knees together. Feel the stretch in the front of the right thigh. Hold for 6-8 seconds, repeat both sides.

12 Calf stretch   *Gastrocnemius*

Assume the correct posture check position. Take one heel behind you. The front knee is bent, knee is above the ankle and the rear leg is straight, push through the rear heel to the floor. Keep the hips and shoulders square and check that the rear toe is facing forward not out to the side. Feel the stretch in the top of the calf muscle in the straight leg. Hold for 6-8 seconds, repeat on the other leg.

13 Back of thigh stretch

Hamstring

Assume your correct posture check position. Bend your left supporting leg slightly, place your right foot flat to the floor in front of the body keeping the leg straight. Lean forwards slightly keeping the chest lifted and the stomach pulled in. Support yourself by placing your hands on the left thigh, feel the stretch all behind the right thigh. Hold for 6-8 seconds, repeat other leg.

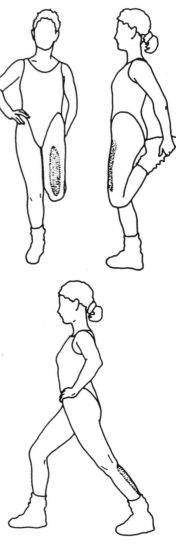

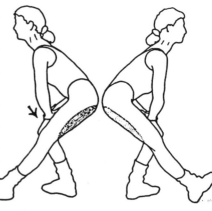

14 Lunge *Adductors*
Assume correct posture check position, then take the feet a good distance apart turning the toes out slightly to 45°. Bend the right knee, the knee should be in line with the ankle. This straightens the left leg. You should feel a comfortable stretch in the inner thigh. Keep the shoulders and hips square. Hold for 6-8 seconds, repeat other side.

15 Side stretch
   Latissimus Dorsi & Obliques
Assume correct posture check position. Place one hand on your hip and take the other arm outstretched over the head. Feel a comfortable stretch all along the side of the body. Keep the shoulders and hips facing forward. Remember the knees should be slightly bent and the stomach pulled in. Breathe out as you hold the stretch position. Hold for 6/8 seconds, repeat other side.

16 Upper back & shoulder stretch *Trapezius and Deltoids*
Assume correct posture check position. Clasp the hands together and extend the arms in front at chest height, pull the stomach in. Feel a comfortable stretch all through the shoulders and the upper back. Drop the head to increase the stretch through the neck. Hold for 6/8 seconds.

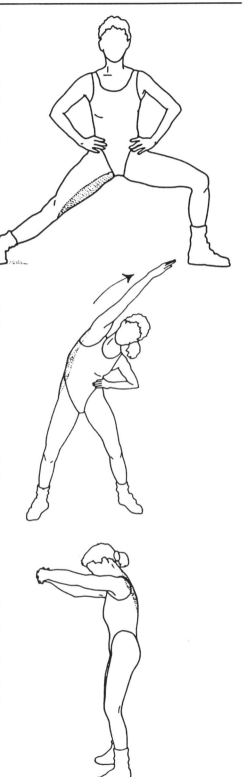

17 Standing chest stretch   *Pectorals*
Assume the correct posture check position.   Clasp your hands
together behind you, squeeze the shoulder blades together as you lift
the hands slightly away from the body.   Feel the stretch all across the
chest.   Hold for 6/8 seconds.

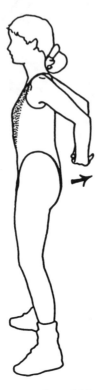

*With all these stretches you should be aware of a mild tension in the
indicated muscles.   DO NOT force or bounce any of the stretches –
they should not be uncomfortable.*

*When you first start stretching you may only want to hold the
position for 6 counts and build up to 8 counts.*

*Always remember to breathe normally, don't hold your breath as you
hold the stretch position.*

TONING EXERCISES

18a Lying side leg raise outer thigh   *Abductors*
Lie on your side with both hips facing forward. Keep the bottom leg bent behind you for extra balance and one hand infront of you to stop you rolling backwards. Breathing normally lift and lower the extended top leg slowly. Keep the knee and toe facing forward. You should feel this exercise all along your outer thigh, check that your leg position does not alter as just a slight realignment of the leg will work the front of the thigh instead of the side. Do 2 sets of 8 repetitions on each leg.

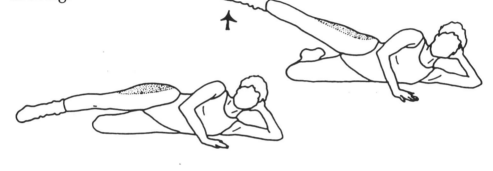

18b Standing side leg raise
Abductors
This standing leg raise works the same muscles. Use a chair or wall for support, make sure the supporting leg is slightly bent and keep the back straight. The knee and toe face forwards when raising the leg out to the side to ensure you use the correct muscles. Do 2 sets of 8 repetitions on each leg, rest between sets if you want to. To increase the intensity of these exercises add to the number of repetitions 3 sets of 8 repetitions.

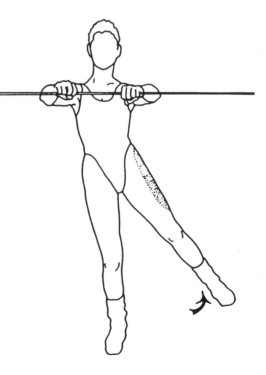

19a Lying inner thigh raise   *Adductors*

Lie on your side.   Extend the lower leg, bring the top leg over the bottom leg so the knee rests gently on the floor in front of you.   Lift and lower the extended bottom leg smoothly.   Remember to keep the knee and toe facing forward.

This exercise can be done slightly faster as the leg can only be raised a small amount due to the limited range of movement.   You will feel this exercise in the inner thigh of the lower leg.   Do 2 sets of 12 repetitions.   To increase the intensity add an extra 1 set of 12 repetitions.

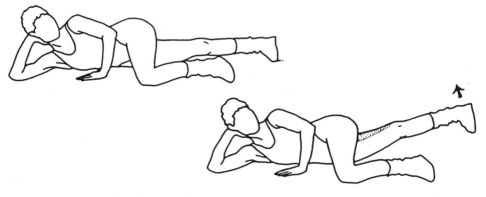

19b Alternative inner thigh raise   *Adductors*

To increase the resistance of this exercise place the heel of the top leg in front onto the extended lower leg. Lift and lower the extended leg smoothly. Place one hand on the floor in front of you for support and to prevent you tipping forwards. Do 2 sets of 12 repetitions.

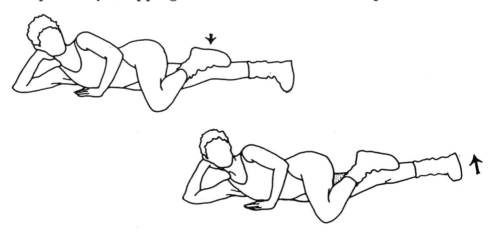

20a Lying bottom & thigh raise *Gluteals & Hamstring*
 Lie face down on the floor. Keep the hips pushed into the floor all
the time. Flex one foot and curl the heel towards the bottom at a 90°
angle. Lift and lower the leg smoothly towards the ceiling squeezing
the bottom as you do so. You should feel this exercise in the back of
the thigh and bottom. If you feel discomfort in the lower back stop,
try an alternative. Do 2 sets of 12 repetitions. This exercise can also
be performed slightly faster.

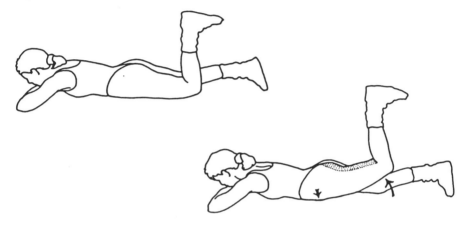

20b Alternate bottom & thigh raise *Gluteals & Hamstring*
You can do this exercise on your elbows and knees. Keep the head
low, the stomach pulled in and the back flat. Flex one foot, bend the
knee at 90° then push the leg upwards towards the ceiling squeezing
the bottom. Then lower to meet the other knee. Try to breathe out
as you push the leg up. Do not take the knee to high or lift the head
as this will make the neck and back arch and may cause pain. Do 2
sets of 8 repetitions on each leg.

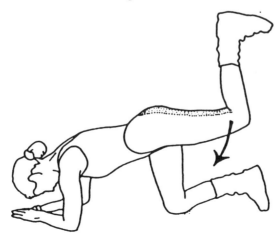

21a Hamstring curl *Hamstring*

Lie face down onto the floor keep the hips pushed down onto the floor. Flex one foot and curl the heel in towards the bottom. Breathe out as you bring the heel in. To make this exercise effective you must squeeze the bottom and thigh as you curl the heel in. To make this exercise harder place the opposite heel over the bottom leg. Then curl in the lower heel with the weight of the top leg pushing down on the bottom leg to increase the resistance. Do 2 sets of 8 repetitions.

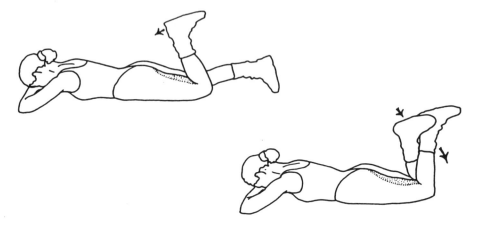

21b Alternative hamstring curl *Hamstring*

Position yourself onto your elbows and knees, your head stays low. Keep the stomach pulled in and the back flat. Raise the leg so the knee is level with the hip, bend the knee curling the heel in towards the bottom. Keep the movement slow and controlled, feel this exercise in the bottom and back of the thigh. Do 2 sets of 8 repetitions with each leg. Increase the intensity by adding a further set of 8 repetitions.

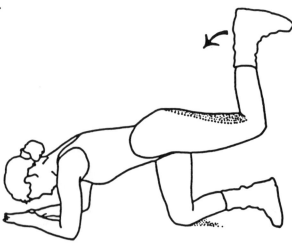

22a Thigh raise
Quadricep & Hip Flexor

Lying back with your knees bent supporting yourself with your elbows, push the hands under your lower back for extra support if you wish. Extend one leg in front of you keeping the leg straight, lift and lower it slowly. The leg only needs to be raised to the height of the opposite knee. You will feel this exercise in the front of the thigh as you raise the leg. Do 2 sets of 8 repetitions. For added resistance place your hand on the thigh you are lifting, push down gently as the leg is raised.

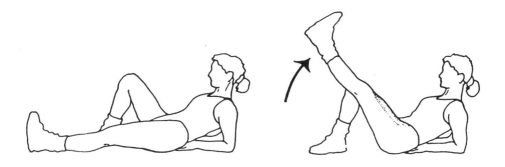

22b Standing thigh raise
Quadricep & Hip Flexor

Stand tall with the stomach pulled in, use a chair or wall for support. Keep the supporting leg slightly bent. Extend one leg in front keeping it straight lift and lower it slowly. Keep the movement controlled, do not swing the leg, feel the exercise in the front of the thigh. Do 2 sets of 8 repetitions with each leg.

To increase the intensity add a further set of 8 repetitions.

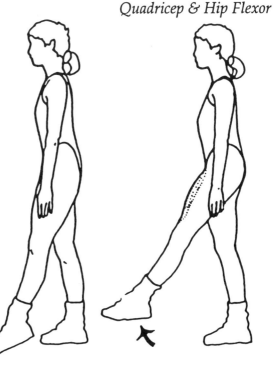

23a Inner thigh squeeze   *Adductors*

Lie down with your lower back pushed firmly down to the ground. Bring the knees in towards the chest. Keeping the heels together open and close the knees, keep the movement controlled. Feel this exercise in the inner thigh. Do 2 sets of 8 repetitions. To increase the intensity do a further set of 8 repetitions, increase the resistance by placing your hands on the outside of the knees and push against the hands as you squeeze the knees together.

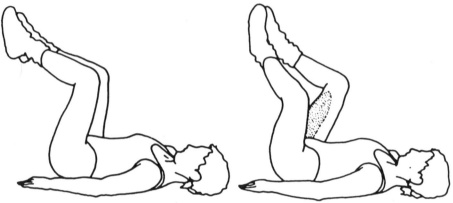

23b Alternative inner thigh squeeze   *Adductors*

This alternative is more difficult. Lying down place your hands under your bottom to give extra support to your back, extend the legs into the air keeping the knees bent over the chest. Open and close the legs keeping the movement slow and controlled, keep the stomach pulled in. Feel this exercise in the inner thigh. Do 2 sets of 8 repetitions.

If you experience any pain in your lower back then please only do exercise 23a.

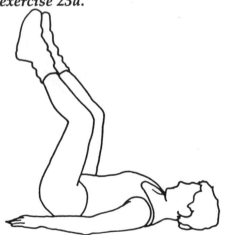 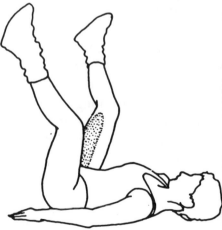

24 Knees bent leg raise *Abductors & Gluteals*
Lie on your side with the knees bent in front at a 90° angle to the body
and the feet flexed. Place one hand on the floor in front of you for
support. Lift and lower the top leg slowly, keeping it at the same
angle as the lower leg. The knee must face forward.
Don't try to lift the leg too high, you should feel this exercise in the
bottom and outer thigh.
Try 2 sets of 8 repetitions with each leg.
Increase the intensity by adding to the repetitions, 3 sets of 8 repetitions.
Increase the resistance by placing your hand on the top leg.

*An alternative would be to perform the exercise with the top leg
straight in line with the hip and shoulder.*

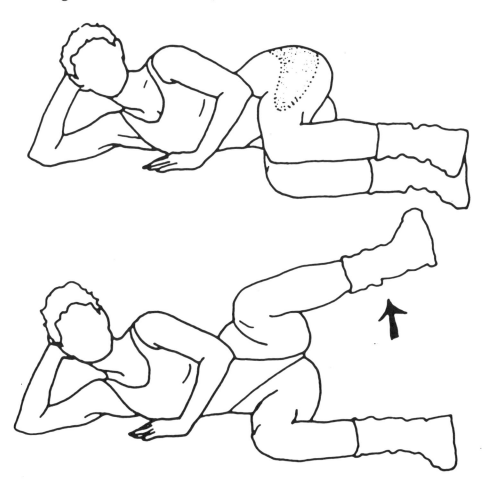

25a Single leg extension   *Quadricep, Hip Flexor*
Lie on your back with your knees bent and feet flat on the floor. Raise
one leg over the body at a right angle. Push through the heel to extend
the leg and then lower. Feel the exercise in the front of the thigh as
the leg extends and flexes. Keep the head and shoulders relaxed and
the lower back pushed into the floor. Do 2 sets of 8 repetitions.
Alternate sets on each leg. Increase intensity by doing exercise 25b.

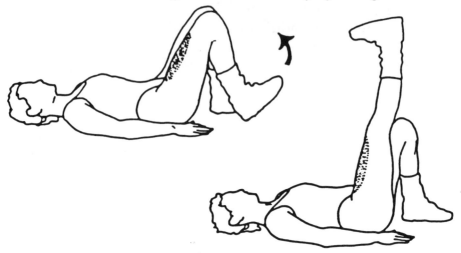

25b Double leg extension   *Quadricep, Hip Flexor & Hamstrings*
In the same position as before bring both knees in towards the chest.
Extend both legs towards the ceiling keeping the knees together and
pushing through the heels. Place both hands under the base of your
spine for extra support of the lower back if you wish. Keep the upper
body relaxed and the stomach pulled in. Do 2 sets of 8 repetitions.

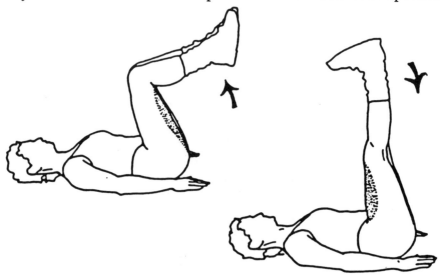

26a Inner thigh raise   *Adductors*

Lie down propped up on the right elbow and with knees bent. Extend the right leg and flex the foot ensuring the foot is turned outwards. Raise and lower the extended right leg no higher than the opposite knee. The toe and knee must face outwards not upwards to ensure you work the inner thigh and not the front of the thigh. Do 2 sets of 8 repetitions with each leg. Be careful not to rock the lower back, keep the movement slow and controlled.

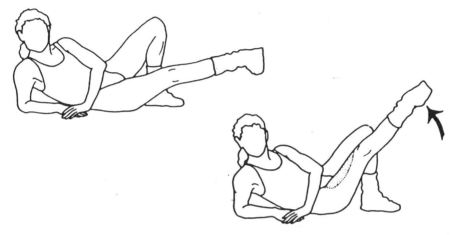

26b Alternative inner thigh raise   *Adductors*

To increase the intensity of this exercise add to the number of repetitions 3 sets of 8 repetitions. To increase the resistance place your hand on the inner thigh of the extended leg and gently push against it as you raise the leg. Keep the back straight and the stomach pulled in. Do 2 sets of 8 repetitions on each leg.

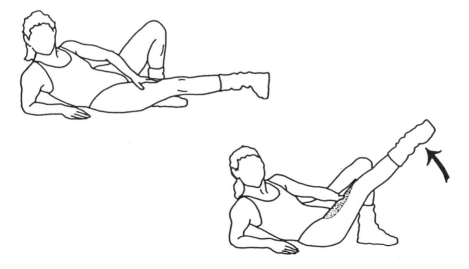

27a Bottom squeeze   *Adductor & Gluteals*

Lying on the floor with your back pushed into the floor, pull the stomach in and tilt the pelvis slightly upwards. Keep the knees and feet together squeeze and release the bottom simultaneously pressing the knees together. Keep the hips still. This is only a small movement and you should feel this exercise in the bottom and the inner thigh. Do 2 sets of 8 repetitions.

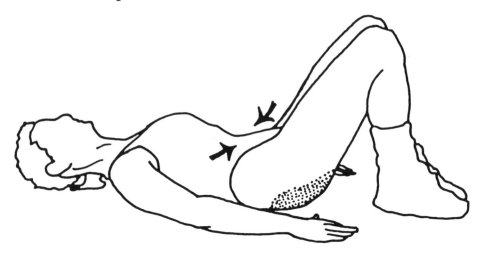

27b Alternative bottom squeeze   *Adductor & Gluteals*

In the same position as 27a raise the back off the floor, support yourself on your shoulders and upper back. Keeping the knees and toes together squeeze and release the bottom as before. Keep the movement small and keep the hips still and the back straight. Do not rock the hips as you do this exercise. If you experience any pain/ discomfort in the lower back please go back to no. 27a. Do 2 sets of 8 repetitions. Increase the intensity by doing a further set of 8 repetitions.

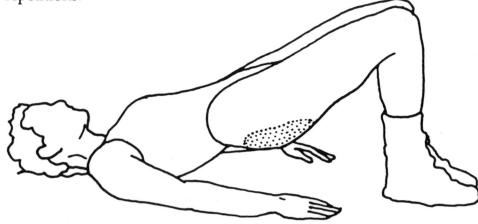

28a Side knee raise   *Abductor & Gluteals*

Position yourself onto your elbows and knees, keep the head low. The knees should be hip width apart for balance. To ensure your back stays flat pull the stomach in, lift and lower the knee slowly to the side without lifting the knee too high. Keep the torso still. Feel this exercise in the bottom and outer thigh. Do 2 sets of 8 repetitions.

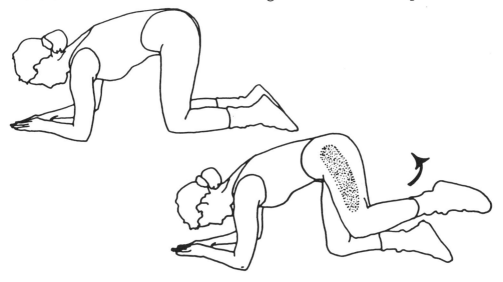

28b Alternative side knee raise   *Abductor & Gluteals*

An alternative position is on your hands and knees. Keeping the knees hip width apart. The hands should be directly beneath the shoulders. Lift and lower the knee to the side as before. Being careful not to swing and tip the shoulder as you lift the knee. Do 2 sets of 8 repetitions. Increase the intensity by adding a further set of repetitions.

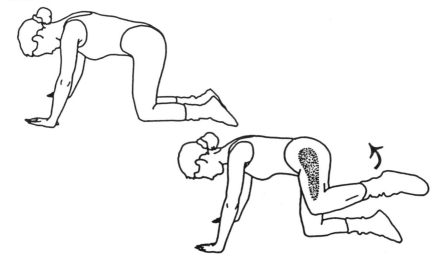

COOLDOWN STRETCHES

29 Standing quad stretch   *Quadricep*
See 'Warm Up' stretch no. 1. Assume the correct posture check
position. Bend the left supporting leg slightly. Draw the right heel
in towards the bottom, holding the foot near the ankle, not curling the
toes. Keep the hips parallel and knees together. Feel the stretch in
the front of the thigh. Push the hip forward to increase the stretch.
Hold for 10-12 seconds, repeat on the other leg.

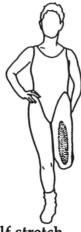 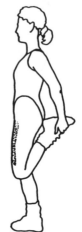

30 Standing calf stretch   *Gastrocnemius*
Assume the correct posture check position, take one heel behind you.
The front leg is bent and the rear leg is straight, push through the back
heel to the floor. Keep the shoulders and hips parallel. Check the rear
toe is facing *forwards* not out to the side as this can alter the muscle
group you are aiming to stretch. Feel the stretch in the top of the calf
muscle. Hold for 10-12 seconds and repeat on the other side.

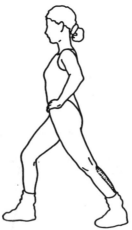

31 Inner thigh stretch   *Adductors*

Sit on the floor bringing the soles of the feet together. Hold the ankles and press the knees down with your elbows until you feel a comfortable stretch in the inner thigh. To increase this stretch part the legs making sure the knees and toes are facing upwards. Keeping the back straight place your hands either behind your bottom or out infront of the body. Feel the stretch all along the inner thigh. Do not force this position. Hold for 10-20 seconds.

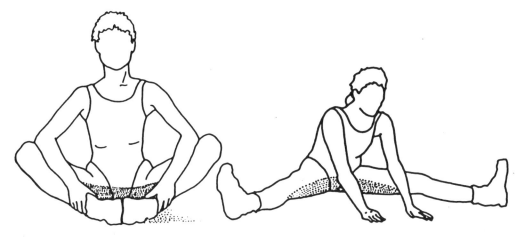

32 Back of thigh stretch   *Hamstring*

Lie on your back with the knees bent, feet flat on the floor. Draw the right knee into the chest then gradually extend the leg supporting it by holding behind the calf or thigh. The leg does not have to be straight, just extend it until you feel a comfortable stretch behind the right thigh. Try to relax the upper body and breathe regularly throughout. Hold for 10-20 seconds. Repeat with other leg.

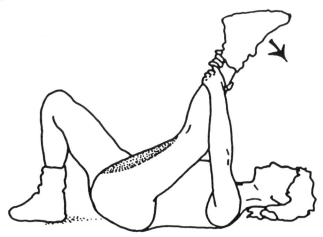

33 Bottom stretch   *Gluteals*

Lie on your back with knees bent and feet flat on the floor. Place the right ankle over the left knee, keeping the right knee pushed away from you. Then draw the left leg towards the chest by clasping your hands together behind the left thigh. This creates a comfortable stretch all around the bottom, hip and thigh area in the right hand side. Hold for 10-12 seconds. Repeat other side.

You may feel this stretch without needing to lift the leg towards the chest.

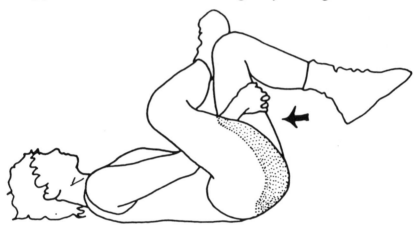

34 Side stretch   *Latissimus Dorsi & Obliques*

Sitting crossed legged, place one hand behind you on the floor. Extend the other arm above you and reach over your head to feel a stretch all along the side of the body. Be careful not to roll sideways and do not lift the bottom off the floor. Hold for 10/12 seconds, repeat on the other side.

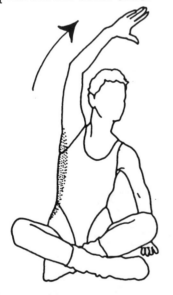
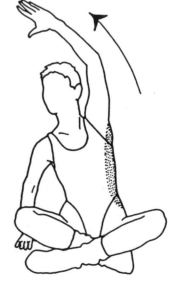

35 Chest stretch   *Pectorals*

Sitting crossed legged clasp the hands together behind you and squeeze the shoulder blades together. Lift the hands slightly away from the body until you feel a comfortable stretch across the chest. Do not force the position and be careful not to arch the back. Hold for 10-12 seconds.

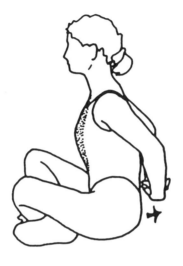

36 Upper back stretch   *Trapezius & Deltoid*

Sitting crossed legged, clasp the hands together and extend the arms in front at chest height. Breathe out as you push the hands away to feel a comfortable stretch across the upper back and shoulders. Drop the head slightly to increase the stretch in the neck area. Keep the stomach pulled in. Hold for 10-12 seconds.

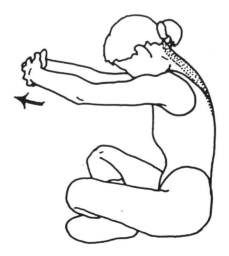

FLATTEN YOUR

STOMACH

WARM UP EXERCISES

1 Shoulder rolls

Assume correct posture check position. Bring the shoulders forward, lift them up and rotate them backwards. Keep the movement slow and controlled. This promotes a feeling of loosening up the shoulder joint. Repeat this 4 times then rotate the shoulders forward 4 times.

2 Head side to side

Assume correct posture check position. With the shoulders down and relaxed, look to your right shoulder, (not over the shoulder) just enough so that your chin is level with your shoulder. Then look to the left shoulder. Repeat 4 times each side. Always face forwards and then turn the head, this gently eases out the neck. *Never* swing from side to side.

3 Side bends

Assume correct posture check position. With the right arm outstretched reach away from the side of the body, simultaneously lifting the elbow of the left arm to shoulder height. The upper body reaches to the right hand side creating a stretch all along the left hand side of the body. Keep the hips and shoulders facing forwards, slowly return to the centre before repeating. Don't swing. Repeat 4 times each side.

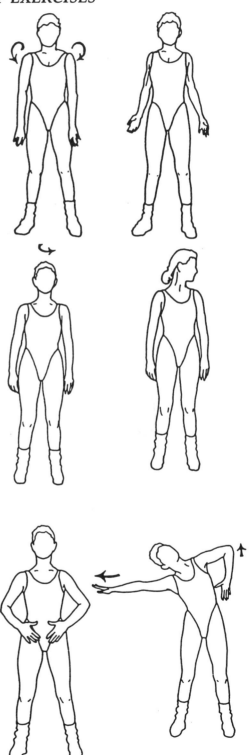

4 Hip circles

Assume correct posture check position. Circle the hips keeping the stomach pulled in. Be careful not to arch the back. Keep the movement slow and controlled. This creates a feeling of 'loosening up' in the lower back. Keep the knees soft and the upper body still. Repeat 4 circles in each direction.

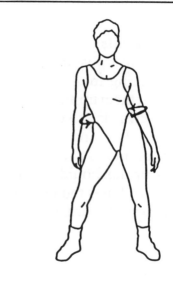

5 Knee bends

Take the feet a good distance apart with the feet turned out slightly at 45°. Keeping the stomach pulled in, the back straight and pelvis tilted forwards, bend and straighten the legs. Be sure not to lock out the knees as you come up. The knees go out over the toes and do not face forward. Do not bend too far as this is only a warm up exercise. Repeat 8 times. Then repeat 8 times adding the arms reaching down and pulling the elbows up to chest height.

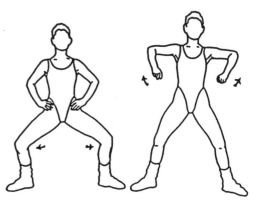

6 Marches

Assume correct posture check position. Bring the feet together and march on the spot. Do not stamp the feet. Keep the back straight and the stomach pulled in. Stand tall. Swing the arms and lift the knees a little higher to add some effort. Repeat 16 times.

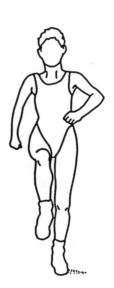

7 Waist twist

Assume correct posture check position. Place your hands on your shoulders and turn your upper body to the right hand side keeping your hips facing forwards. Face back to the centre and click your fingers before turning to the left hand side. Keep your stomach pulled in flat and feel this exercise in the waist. Always come to centre before changing direction. Do not swing. Keep the knees soft. Repeat 4 times each side.

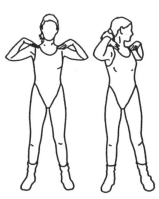

8 Rib isolation

Assume correct posture check position. Extend the arms at shoulder height. Move the upper body to the right hand side and back to the centre isolating the ribs and upper body. Keep the hips and lower body quite still. The knees remain soft. Pull the stomach in flat. The movement is from side to side not pushing the chest forward. Always keep the movement controlled. Feel this exercise in the waist area. Do 8 repetitions to alternate sides.

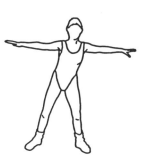

9 Swing step

Take the feet wide apart and step from one foot to the other. Bend the knees through the middle as you transfer your weight. At the same time swing arms at shoulder height. The more effort you put into this exercise by taking larger steps and bending more in the middle the warmer you become. Repeat for 8 swings.

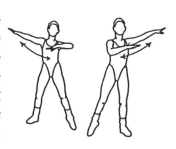

10 Swing step & heel raise

Repeat as above, at the same time lift alternate heels in towards the bottom. Make sure your supporting leg is always bent. Don't lock out the knees. Repeat 8 times. Now repeat exercises 9 and 10.

You should now feel warmer and ready to stretch, if you do not please repeat exercise 10

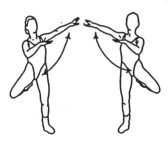

WARM UP STRETCHES

11 Front thigh   *Quadricep*
Assume correct posture check position. Bend the left supporting leg slightly and draw the opposite heel in towards the bottom holding the foot near the ankle *(not curling the toes)*. Keep the hips square and pushed forward and the knees together. Feel the stretch in the front of the right thigh. Hold for 6-8 seconds. Repeat both sides.

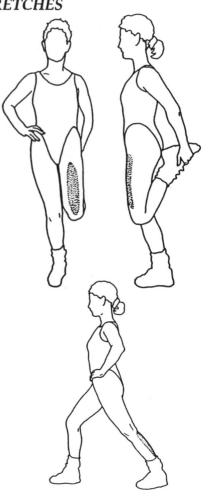

12 Calf stretch   *Gastrocnemius*
Assume correct posture check position. Place one heel behind you. The front knee is bent, knee is over the ankle and the rear leg is straight. Push through the rear heel to the floor. Keep the hips and shoulders square and check that the rear toe is facing forward not out to the side. Feel the stretch at the top of the calf muscle in the straight leg. Hold for 6-8 seconds, repeat on the other leg.

13 Back of thigh stretch   *Hamstring*
Assume correct posture check position. Bend your left supporting leg slightly, place your right foot flat to the floor in front of the body, keeping the leg straight. Lean forwards slightly keeping the chest lifted and the stomach pulled in. Support yourself by placing your hands on the left thigh. Feel the stretch all behind the right thigh. Hold for 6-8 seconds, repeat other leg.

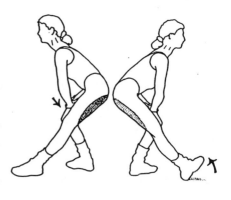

14 Tricep stretch *Tricep*
Assume correct posture check position.
Place the right hand over your head with
the finger tips between your shoulder
blades. The left hand rests gently on the
right elbow to ease the arm into position. If
you feel uncomfortable in this position place
the left arm on the arm in front of the body
rather than above as shown in the diagram.
Hold for 8 seconds. Feel the stretch in back
of the upper arm. Repeat other side.

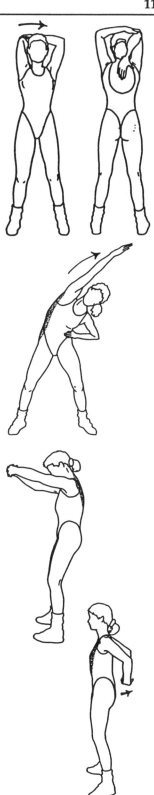

15 Side stretch *Latissimus dorsi & obliques*
Assume correct posture check position.
Place one hand on your hip and take the
other arm outstretched over the head. Feel
a comfortable stretch all along the side of
the body. Keep the shoulders and hips
facing forward. Remember the knees
should be slightly bent and the stomach
pulled in. Breathe out as you hold the
stretch position. Hold for 6-8 seconds.
Repeat other side.

16 Upper back *Trapezius and deltoids*
Assume correct posture check position.
Clasp hands together and extend the arms
in front at chest height, pulling the stomach
in. Feel a comfortable stretch all through
the shoulders and the upper back. Drop the
head to increase the stretch through the
neck. Hold for 6-8 seconds.

17 Chest stretch *Pectorals*
Assume correct posture check position.
Clasp your hands together behind you,
squeeze the shoulder blades together as
you lift the hands slightly away from the
body. Be careful not to lock out the elbows.
Feel the stretch all across the chest. Hold
for 6-8 seconds.

TONING EXERCISES

18a Curl up   *Rectus abdominus*

Lie on the floor with the knees bent and hip width apart. Place one hand on your thigh and one hand behind the ear. Raise the head and shoulders keeping the stomach flat and back pressed into the floor. Slide the other hand along the thigh and over the knee. As you curl up breathe out. Do 2 sets of 8 repetitions.

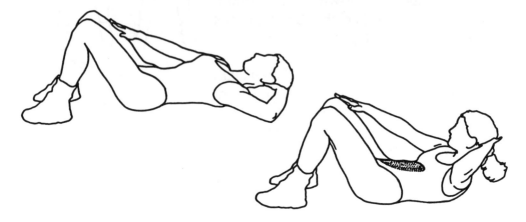

18b Alternative curl up   *Rectus abdominus*

Lie on the floor with the knees bent. Feet flat on the floor hip width apart. Place both hands behind the ears. Pull the stomach in flat and curl the head and shoulders up from the floor to feel the adominals working. Keep the back pressed down firmly . Be careful not to pull on the neck. Just let the head rest in the hands. Breathe out as you lift. Keep the movement slow and controlled. Do 2 sets of 8 repetitions.

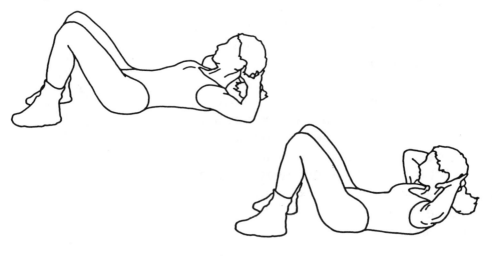

19a Oblique curl up
Obliques

Lie on the floor with knees bent, feet flat on the floor hip width apart. Place the right hand behind the right ear. Keeping the stomach flat curl the shoulders off the floor and twist the left shoulder gently to the right hand side leaning on your right elbow. The left hand reaches to the outside of the right knee. Keep the stomach flat. Remember to breathe out on the effort. Do 2 sets of 8 repetitions alternate sides.

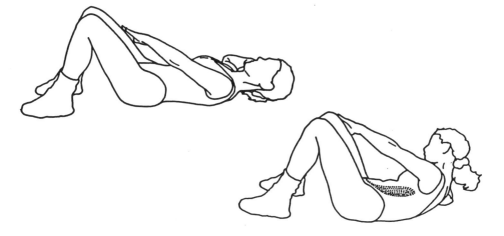

19b Alternative oblique curl up
Obliques

Lie on the floor with knees bent hip width apart. Place both hands beside your ears. Contract the stomach, curl up and twist the left shoulder towards the right knee, keeping the right elbow on the floor for support. Curl up and down but do not allow the head to touch the floor. Between repetitions keep the lower back pressed down into the floor. Exhale as you curl up. Do 2 sets of 8 repetitions

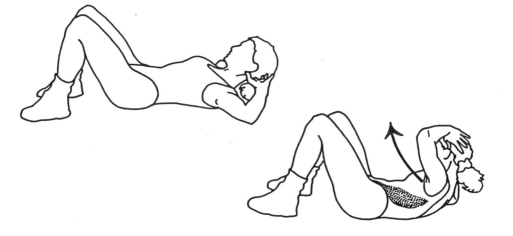

20a Tricep dip   *Tricep*
Sit on the floor with the knees bent and feet flat on the floor. Place your hands behind you beneath the shoulders with the finger tips facing forwards parallel with your legs and feet. Lean backwards slowly bending the elbows then push up extending the arms – be careful not to snap out the elbows. Feel this exercise in the back of the upper arm. Keep the stomach pulled in.   Do 2 sets of 8 repetitions.

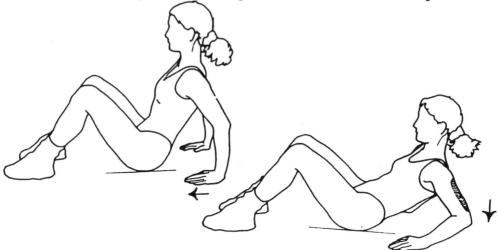

20b Raised tricep dip   *Tricep*
In the same position as above raise the bottom from the floor. Keep the finger tips facing forwards. Bend and extend the arms working the back of the upper arm. Be sure to bend the arms. Do not just lift and lower the bottom. Rest as necessary. Do not snap out the elbows as you extend the arms. Do stretch No 14 (p 21) to relieve tension as necessary.   Do 2 sets of 8 repetitions.

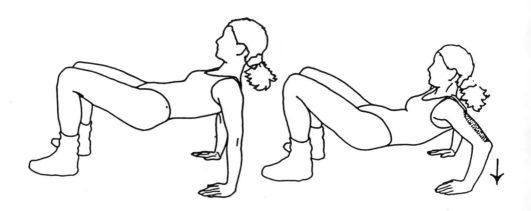

21a Crossed curl up   *Rectus abdominus*

Lie on the floor with the knees bent, feet flat on the floor hip width apart. Cross the arms over the chest and contract the stomach pressing the lower back firmly down. Curl the head and shoulders up and then down. Remember to breathe and keep the stomach really flat. Try not to let the head fall back between repetitions. Do 2 sets of 8 repetitions.

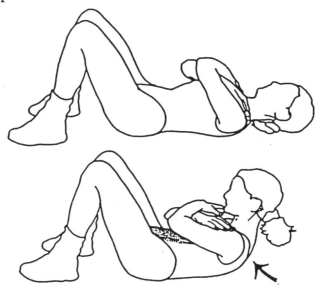

21b Alternative crossed curl up   *Rectus abdominus*

To vary this exercise and increase the intensity you can lift for 2 counts and lower for 2 counts. Try to hold the uppermost position briefly before curling down. Remember to keep the chin forward over the chest to prevent any tension in the neck. Keep the stomach really flat. The movement should be smooth and controlled. Breathe out on the effort. Feel this exercise really working the stomach. Do 2 sets of 8 repetitions.

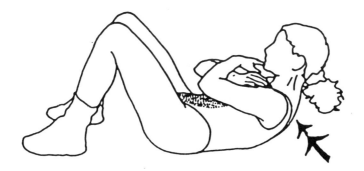

22a Oblique twist   *Obliques*

Lie on the floor with knees bent. Place right ankle over left knee. Right hand rests behind right ear & elbow stays on the floor for support. Left hand reaches round right knee as you raise head and shoulder and twist the torso towards right knee. Keep right knee open – do not pull on it, stomach flat and back pressed down. Keep the movement slow and controlled – feel this exercise in waist area. As you return to the starting position do not let head fall back to the floor. Exhale on the effort. Do 2 sets of 8 repetitions each side.

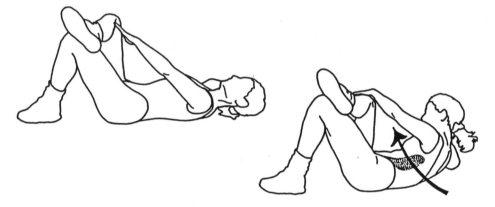

22b Alternative oblique twist   *Obliques*

In the same position as before alter arm position, place both hands behind ears. Keep neck relaxed and passive. Curl shoulders off the floor and twist left shoulder to right knee keeping right elbow on the floor. Try to hold at the uppermost position briefly before curling down. Keep lower back pressed into floor. Feel this exercise in the waist area. Rest as necessary. Do 2 sets of 8 repetitions each side.

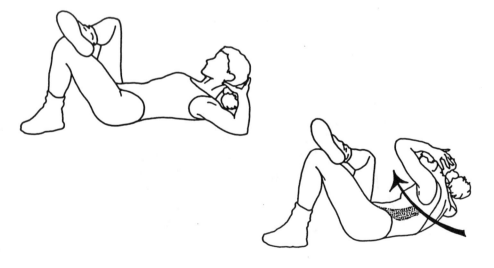

23a Box press up   *Pectorals and triceps*
On your hands and knees – knees are hip width apart. Place hands beneath shoulders approximately shoulder distance apart with the finger tips facing forward, hips directly over the knees. Pull the stomach in and tilt the pelvis forward to support a flat back. Lower body towards the floor bending arms until nose is nearly touching the floor. Ensure back stays flat. Do not snap out elbows as you extend arms. Keep the movement controlled. Breathe out as you push up. Do 2 sets of 8 repetitons.

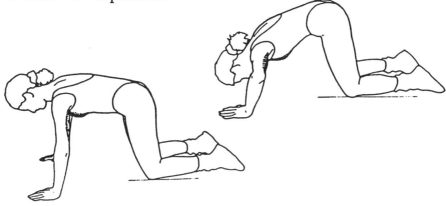

23b Three quarter press up   *Pectorals and triceps*
Assume above position, walk hands further in front keeping them shoulder width apart and shifting body weight forwards, hips now further in front of knees. Keep stomach pulled in. Remember the pelvic tilt and keep back flat. Lower body towards the floor bending elbows. Push up, extending arms but not locking out elbows. Rest as necessary. Breathe out as you push up. Do 2 sets of 8 repetitions.

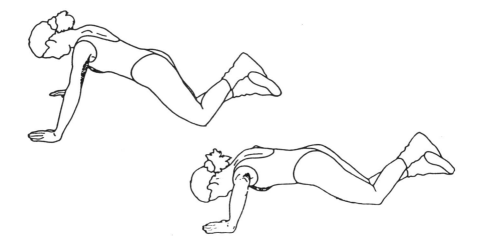

24a Crunches   *Rectus abdominus*

Lie on the floor and bring the knees over the hips creating a right angle
to the floor. Rest the hands behind the ears or across the chest. Keep
the stomach pulled in and the lower back pressed into the floor. Curl
the head and shoulders off the floor. Only lift as far as you can whilst
still keeping the stomach flat. Ensure the knees stay over the hips.
Remember to breathe out as you curl up. Rest as necessary. Do 2 sets
of 8 repetitions.

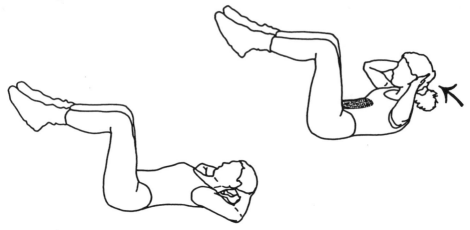

24b Alternative crunches   *Rectus abdominus*

To vary this exercise and increase the intensity without altering the
position you can curl up for 2 counts and lower for 2 counts. Ensure
that the knees stay over the hips to keep the lower back pressed into
the floor. Keep the stomach flat and feel this exercise throughout the
abdominal region. Keep the movement smooth and controlled and
try to hold the uppermost positon briefly before curling down.
Exhale on the effort. Do 2 sets of 8 repetitions.

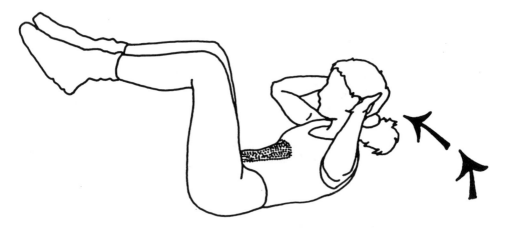

25a Crunch with oblique twist *Obliques*

Lie on the floor with the knees raised over the hips, hands resting behind the ears. Keep the neck relaxed and passive. Contract the stomach, raise the head and shoulders and twist the left shoulder towards the right knee then lower, not allowing the head to touch the floor between repetitions. Keep the stomach flat. Feel this exercise in the waist. Do 2 sets of 8 repetitions on each side.

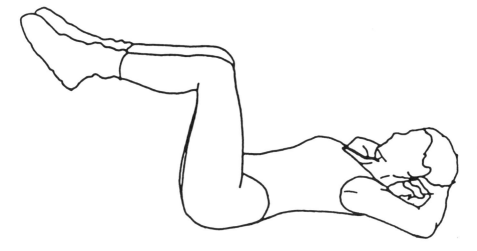

25b Alternative crunch with oblique twist *Obliques*

Vary this exercise position and increase the intensity whilst remaining in the same starting position. Contract the stomach and raise the head and shoulders. Twist the torso leading with the left shoulder towards the right knee. Raise for 2 counts and curl down for 2 counts holding the uppermost positon briefly. Remember to exhale as you curl up and try not to let the head touch the floor between repetitions. Do 2 sets of 8 repetitions on alternate sides.

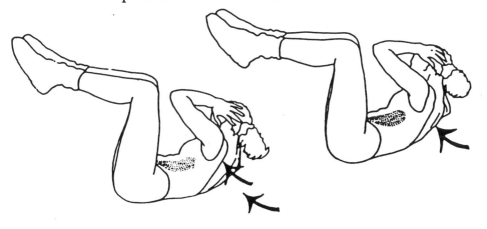

26a Lower back extension   *Erector spinae*

Lie face down on the floor with elbows bent at shoulder level and hands palms down on either side of the head near the face. The legs are straight, with feet on the floor. Keep facing downwards, do not look forward. This protects the neck and prevents hyperextension. Keeping the head and neck still, raise upper body, still keeping hands and elbows on the floor. Hips must stay pressed to the floor. Keep looking down. Only lift as far as is comfortable. Feel this exercise in lower back. Keep the movement slow and controlled. Rest between sets as necessary. Do 2 sets of 8 repetitions.

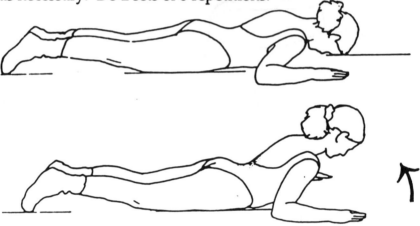

26b Alternative lower back extension   *Erector spinae*

Alter the position by placing hands behind you on your bottom. Whilst facing downwards raise upper body a few inches off the floor and then lower gently. Keep the movement slow and controlled, not jerky. Keep hips and feet on the floor. Breathe normally, rest as necessary. Do 2 sets of 8 repetitions.

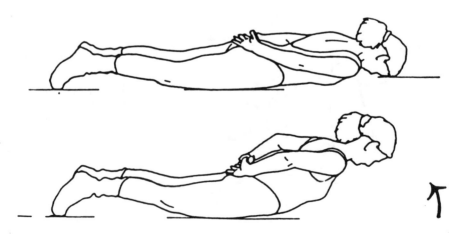

27a Reverse curl *Rectus abdominus*

Lie on the floor and bring knees into chest, cross ankles and let knees separate. Extend arms and place hands above head, palms upwards. Keep feet in towards the bottom. Having knees over chest/stomach helps to keep lower back into the ground. Squeeze and contract stomach into your back and your back into the floor. This tilts the pelvis forward and shortens the distance between ribs and hips. Your legs may move slightly. Concentrate on squeezing stomach not swinging legs. Breathe normally. Rest as necessary. Do 2 sets of 8 repetitions.

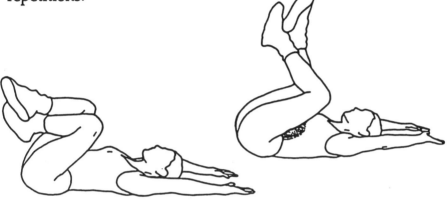

27b Alternative reverse curl *Rectus abdominus*

Lie down on the floor and extend legs above you. Keep knees slightly bent over stomach, cross ankles. Squeeze stomach into your back and your back into floor. As abdominals contract your pelvis will tilt slightly forward causing legs to lift slightly. Concentrate on squeezing abdominals, not swinging the legs. This is a very subtle movement. Imagine you are shortening the distance between navel and pubic bone. Feel this exercise in lower abdominal region. Remember to breathe. Do 2 sets of 8 repetitions. Place the hands beside you if you prefer.

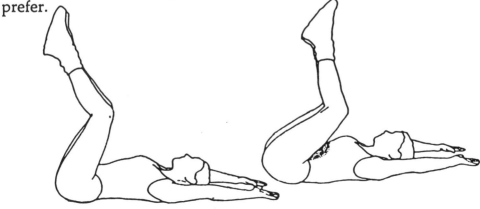

28a Oblique twist with leg extension   *Oblique and hip flexors*

Lie on floor with knees bent, place hands gently behind ears. Keep right foot flat on the floor and extend left leg so that knees are level. Keeping lower back pressed down and stomach flat, curl up head and shoulder and twist torso towards left hand side simultaneously tucking left knee towards chest and meeting right elbow. Curl down and extend leg. Remember to keep head slightly away from the floor between repetitions. Do not pull on head and neck. Feel this exercise in waist and top of thigh. Do 2 sets of 8 repetitions each side.

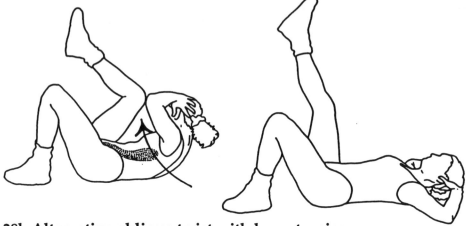

28b Alternative oblique twist with leg extension

Oblique and hip flexors

To vary this exercise lower extended leg position. Instead of raising leg, extend leg, pushing through heel. Make sure other leg is bent with foot flat on floor to support lower back. As above, curl up and cross opposite shoulder to opposite knee squeezing stomach throughout. Do 2 sets of 8 repetitions.

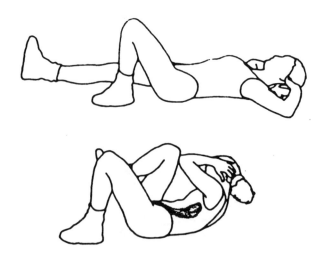

29a Upper back exercise *Rhomboids*
Kneel on the left knee with the right knee in front of you at a right angle. Lean forward so that your chest rests on your knee. Your shoulders must stay facing forward. Keep looking down to ensure your neck stays in line with your spine. To keep the shoulders square rest your left hand on the floor. Your right hand is down by your side making a fist. Bring back your right hand moving your elbow upwards until it is level with your shoulder. Take the arm back to the starting position and repeat. Be careful not to twist the torso, the chest and hips must stay facing downwards squarely. Rest as necessary. Feel this exercise in the upper back. To increase the effectiveness try using a small hand weight such as a tin of beans. Do 2 sets of 8 repetitions on each side.

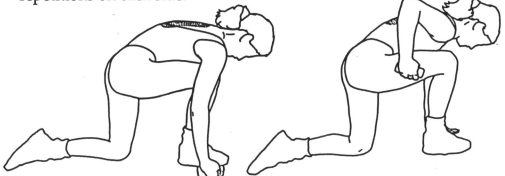

29b Alternative upper back exercise *Rhomboids*
Start in a full press up position, hands shoulder distance apart directly beneath the shoulders. Feet are hip width apart, the bottom is low, not sticking in the air. Raise the right hand, bending the arm until the elbow is level with the shoulder. Keep both shoulders facing forward and do not twist the torso. Alternate this exercise from right to left. If this is too hard you can put the knees onto the ground making a three quarter press up position. Rest as necessary. Do 2 sets of 8 repetitions, alternate hands.

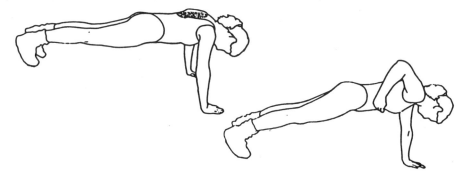

COOLDOWN STRETCHES

30 Standing quad stretch
See *Warm Up* stretch no 1.
Assume the correct posture
check position. Bend the left
supporting leg slightly.
Draw the right heel in towards the bottom, holding
the foot near the ankle, not
curling the toes. Keep the
hips parallel and the knees
together. Feel the stretch in
the front of the thigh. Push
the hip forward to increase
the stretch. Hold for 10-12
seconds, repeat on the other
leg.

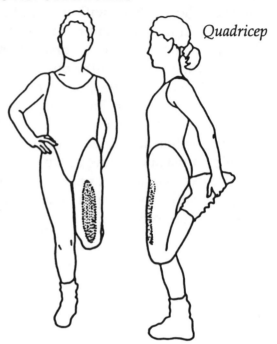

Quadricep

31 Standing calf stretch
Assume the correct posture
check position, take one heel
behind you. The front leg is
bent and the rear leg is
straight, push through the
back heel to the floor. Keep
shoulders and hips parallel.
Check the rear toe is facing
forwards not out to the side
as this can alter the muscle
group you are aiming to
stretch in the top of the calf
muscle. Hold for 10-12 seconds and repeat on the other
side.

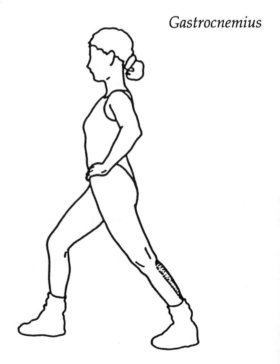

Gastrocnemius

32 Side stretch *Latissimus dorsi and obliques*
Sit crossed legged, place one hand behind you on the floor.
Extend other arm above you and reach over head to feel a stretch
along side of body. Be careful not to roll sideways and do not lift the
bottom off the floor. Hold for 10-12 seconds, repeat on other side.

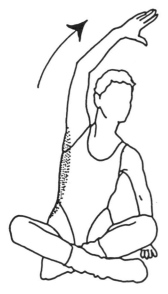 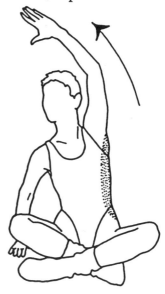

33 Upper back stretch *Trapezius and deltoids*
Sit crossed legged, clasp hands together and extend arms in front at
chest height. Breathe out as you push hands away to feel a comfortable stretch across upper back and shoulders. Drop head slightly
increasing stretch in neck area. Keep stomach pulled in. Hold for 10-
12 seconds.

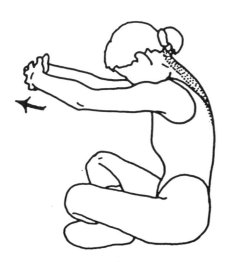

34 Chest stretch   *Pectorals*

Sitting crossed legged clasp hands behind you and squeeze shoulder blades together. Lift hands slightly away from body until you feel a comfortable stretch across the chest. Do not force the position and do not to arch back. Hold for 10-12 seconds.

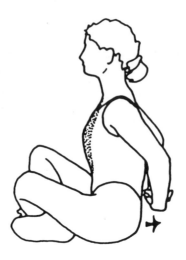

35 Back of thigh stretch   *Hamstring*

Lie on your back with the knees bent, feet flat on the floor. Draw the right knee into the chest then gradually extend the leg supporting it by holding it behind the calf or thigh. The leg does not have to be straight, just extend it until you feel a comfortable stretch behind the right thigh. Try to relax the upper body and breathe regularly throughout. Hold for 10-20 seconds. Repeat with other leg.

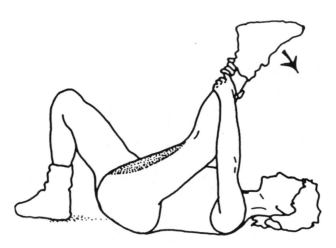

36 Waist stretch   *Obliques*

Lie on the floor with the knees bent, feet flat on the floor. Gently roll your knees over to one side to rest on the floor and take your arms to the opposite side, feel a comfortable stretch in the waist. Hold for 10-12 seconds. Repeat the other side. If you have any discomfort in your lower back then keep your arms on the same side as your knees.

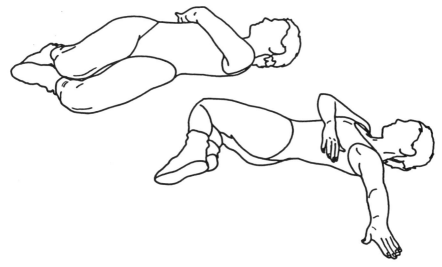

37 Lower back   *Erector sinae and back generally*

Lie on the floor and bring both knees into chest. Clasp hands around knees. Keep head and shoulders relaxed on the ground and gently rock knees from side to side, massaging lower spine. Repeat this a few times.

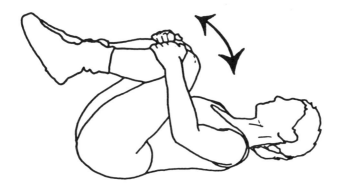

38 Stomach stretch   *Rectus abdominus and generally all over*

Lie flat on the floor with legs and arms outstretched – really reach through finger tips and point your toes to feel a stretch throughout stomach area and generally all over. Hold for 8-10 seconds and repeat.

If you have back problems keep one knee bent with the foot flat to the floor to help support the back

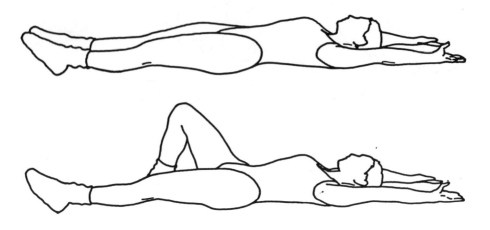

39 Neck relaxation   *Sternocleidomastoid*

Lie on your back with knees bent, feet flat on floor. Gently roll head from side to side to release tension in the neck. Repeat four times.

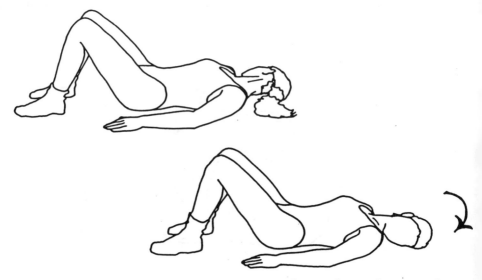

The last 4 stretches/relaxation exercises can be performed at any time between the toning exercises to relieve tension.